EMDR *and the*
Universal Healing Tao

EMDR *and the* Universal Healing Tao

An Energy Psychology Approach to Overcoming Emotional Trauma

Mantak Chia and Doug Hilton

Destiny Books
Rochester, Vermont • Toronto, Canada

Destiny Books
One Park Street
Rochester, Vermont 05767
www.DestinyBooks.com

Destiny Books is a division of Inner Traditions International

Originally published in Thailand in 2014 by Universal Tao Publications under the
title *Taoist Emotional Recycling: Energetic Psychological Approach*

Library of Congress Cataloging-in-Publication Data
Names: Chia, Mantak, 1944- author. | Hilton, Doug, author.
Title: EMDR and the universal healing Tao : an energy psychology approach to
    overcoming emotional trauma / Mantak Chia and Doug Hilton.
Other titles: Taoist emotional recycling energetic psychological approach
Description: Rochester, Vermont : Destiny Books, [2017] | Includes
    bibliographical references and index.
Identifiers: LCCN 2016027588 (print) | LCCN 2016048978 (e-book) |
    ISBN 9781620555514 (paperback) | ISBN 9781620555521 (e-book)
Subjects: LCSH: Psychic trauma—Alternative treatment. | Eye movement
    desensitization and reprocessing. | Qi gong. | Self-help techniques. |
    BISAC: HEALTH & FITNESS / Alternative Therapies. | BODY,
    MIND & SPIRIT / Healing / Energy (Chi Kung, Reiki, Polarity).
Classification: LCC RC552.T7 C45 2017 (print) | LCC RC552.T7 (e-book) |
    DDC 616.85/21—dc23
LC record available at https://lccn.loc.gov/2016027588

Printed and bound in the United States by Versa Press, Inc.

10 9 8 7 6 5 4 3 2 1

Text design and layout by Priscilla Baker
This book was typeset in Garamond Premier Pro with Diotima, Present, and
Futura used as display typefaces
Photographs in chapters 6 through 8 by Sopitnapa Promnon

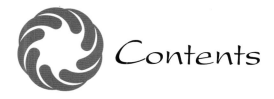

Contents

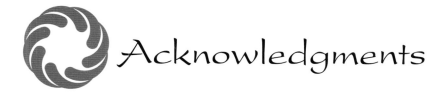 # Acknowledgments

The authors and Universal Healing Tao Publications staff involved in the preparation and production of *EMDR and the Universal Healing Tao* extend our gratitude to the many generations of Taoist masters who have passed on their special lineage, in the form of an unbroken oral transmission, over thousands of years. We thank Taoist Master Yi Eng (One Cloud Hermit) for his openness in transmitting the formulas of Taoist Inner Alchemy.

We offer our eternal gratitude to our parents and teachers for their many gifts to us. Remembering them brings joy and satisfaction to our continued efforts in presenting the Universal Healing Tao system. For their gifts, we offer our eternal gratitude and love. As always, their contribution has been crucial in presenting the concepts and techniques of the Universal Healing Tao.

We wish to thank the thousands of unknown men and women of the Taoist healing arts who developed many of the methods and ideas presented in this book. For their continuous personal encouragement, we wish to thank our fellow Taoists, students, clients, families, and friends who have inspired the writing of this book by their eager desire to understand Taoist Emotional Recycling.

We thank the many contributors essential to this book's final form: the editorial and production staff at Inner Traditions/Destiny Books for their efforts to clarify the text and produce a handsome new edition of the book, and Nancy Yeilding for her line edit of the new edition.

A special thanks goes to our Thai production team for their efforts on the first edition of this book: Hirunyathorn Punsan, Sopitnapa Promnon, Udon Jandee, and Suthisa Chaisarn.

Doug Hilton would like to thank: His wife Ana for all her love and support through the writing process; Master Mantak Chia for all of his knowledge, wisdom, guidance, and support; Dell Graff for introducing him to the field of addictions counseling; Veronica Graff for introducing him to the value of older traditions; Brent Neumann for numerous thought-provoking conversations; Donna Baird for introducing him to EMDR and for continual support; Dr. Sal Mendaglio for introducing him to the concept of polarities; Gerald Hilton for his encouragement and continual reminders of the value of polar opposites; Edward Gutierrez for his wisdom and continual encouragement; Jutta and Walter Kellenberger for their quiet and steady support; Gordon Mah for offering a patient and encouraging ear; Dr. Marshall Wilensky for teaching EMDR to him; Dr. Francine Shapiro for discovering EMDR; Dr. Robert Miller for creating the Feeling-State Addiction Protocol; all the Taoist masters who have contributed to the current knowledge; and the thousands of clients who have shared their wisdom and experience over the years. Special thanks also go to William U. Wei for his patience and diligence during the production process of the original edition.

Putting Taoist Emotional Recycling into Practice

The information presented in this book is based on the authors' personal experience and knowledge of Taoist Emotional Recycling. The practices described in this book have been used successfully for thousands of years by Taoists trained by personal instruction. Readers should not undertake the practices on themselves or others without receiving personal transmission, training, and certification from a certified instructor of Taoist Emotional Recycling, since certain of these practices, if done improperly, may cause injury or result in health problems. This book is intended to supplement individual training by the Universal Healing Tao and to serve as a reference guide for these practices. Anyone who undertakes these practices on the basis of this book alone does so entirely at his or her own risk.

The meditations, practices, and techniques described herein are not intended to be used as an alternative to or substitute for professional medical treatment and care. If any readers are suffering from illnesses based on physical, mental, or emotional disorders, an appropriate professional health care practitioner or therapist should be consulted. Such problems should be corrected before you start Universal Healing Tao training.

Neither the Universal Healing Tao nor its staff and instructors can be responsible for the consequences of any practice or misuse of the information contained in this book. If the reader undertakes any exercise without strictly following the instructions, notes, and warnings, the responsibility must lie solely with the reader.

This book does not attempt to give any medical diagnosis, treatment, prescription, or remedial recommendation in relation to any human disease, ailment, suffering, or physical condition whatsoever.

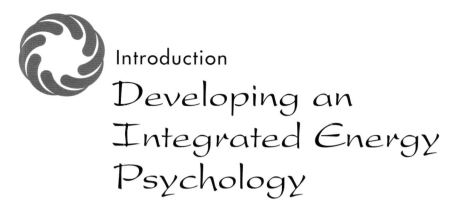

Introduction

Developing an Integrated Energy Psychology

By Doug Hilton

I started training to be a psychotherapist in 1984. Throughout my training I had questions that were never answered. For example, in my first personality theory class the professor told us that most of us were coming to learn about psychology because we had a desire to fix ourselves, not just help other people. That was certainly true for me.

However, as I worked in various areas of the psychology field it did not seem like my mental health or the mental health of my colleagues was significantly improving with experience. I started to wonder if a lack of wellness was characteristic of people who chose counseling as a profession or if it was created or made worse by working in the field. If counselors became unhealthy from working in the field, I wondered how that could happen and what to do to prevent it.

Relatedly, in graduate school I remember being told that there would be times when I would end a day of counseling and feel like I was still wearing the emotions of the clients I had seen that day. The professor told us not to take on the emotions of our clients. He told us we might

1

each need to have our own counselor to talk to so that we could keep those feelings from piling up inside of us and becoming unmanageable. That was the extent of our training on this important aspect of counseling. I had no clue how to detach myself, protect myself, or get rid of the unhealthy effects that I was absorbing from my clients.

I was confused by the emphasis on the mind and the brain in many classical approaches to counseling, when it seems to be common knowledge that our minds and bodies are connected. My clients were continually complaining about physical problems that seemed related to their emotional challenges, but I did not know how to help them. I had even more trouble understanding how issues like addictions and eating disorders were treated primarily by telling people to think differently.

I was surprised at how often clients were not able to resolve the challenges that they faced, and even more shocked at how often they were labeled as having a personality disorder and written off as being beyond help if their progress was not quick and steady. I wondered how my field had become so seemingly complacent.

Then in 2001 I trained in Eye Movement Desensitization and Reprocessing (EMDR), a revolution in the field of counseling. It took a big step toward addressing the cycles and dynamics that challenge us in a practical way. EMDR is a special counseling technique that is now used all over the world to help people put away bad feelings about things that have happened to them in the past that still bother them. It has been especially helpful for treating post-traumatic stress disorder (PTSD) in both soldiers returning from war and in the general population. It does not involve or require much in the way of interpretation, advice, or homework. It recognizes the mind-body connection and works with energy (whether that is officially recognized or not). It has been highly researched and refined over the years into a treatment that provides fast and permanent results for the majority of people who receive the treatment.

HOW EMDR WORKS

EMDR uses sets of bilateral (back-and-forth) stimulation of the senses while the person focuses on key aspects of the issue that need to be addressed. It was originally done with eye movements, which is the origin of the name. However, now it is also done with stimulation to the sense of touch—through tapping on the legs of the client—or hearing—by snapping outside of his or her ears, respectively. An electronic device has even been developed that can produce sensations, moving lights, and sounds to provide the stimulation.

In the EMDR protocol, the counselor introduces the method to the client, and the issue to be worked on is identified and clarified. This is followed by three treatment phases: Desensitization, in which negative feelings and urges are processed away; Positive Installation, which builds up positive beliefs; and the Body Scan, which works on removing any lingering negative physical sensations.

The bottom line is that the procedure works. Once people complete all three phases, the bad feelings or urges do not come back. It works very quickly compared to most other existing counseling approaches. The client does not even have to believe in it for it to be effective.

MAKING DYNAMIC CONNECTIONS

Learning EMDR gave me a whole new way to help people, a way that seemed more holistic and less reliant on an exchange between clients and myself. They were healing themselves. I was just guiding them through the process. It felt like I had ended up with an approach that was more clinically satisfying. EMDR produces much quicker and more concrete results. However, because it was discovered by accident, in the training we were never given any definitive explanations of why it works.

In 2004 I went to Tao Garden, the beautiful training center and healing spa that Master Chia created in Thailand. I had received a taste of what he has to offer in San Francisco and was eager to learn more after that. I was fortunate enough to learn about Tao Garden while attending that first training and to be in a position to come for the full summer retreat to learn some more. Like many of the participants at the retreat, I had many unanswered questions about my life and life in general. I found that Master Chia and the Universal Healing Tao system that he organized provided the answers I craved.

When I was in Tao Garden I started to make connections in my mind between the field of psychotherapy and the Chi Kung practices being taught there. I began to get the impression that the meditation I was learning might be doing something similar to what happens with EMDR. Even though my previous experiences of talking about EMDR with people who use a different approach had not been positive, I really wanted to know what Master Chia thought of the technique, so I nervously approached him at the end of one of the meditation classes. When I asked him if he had heard of EMDR he said, "No. What's that?" I was surprised that no one had talked to him about it before. I thought that perhaps there were not that many counselors who had the same kinds of questions that I had.

In a couple of sentences I explained about the bilateral (back-and-forth) stimulation that EMDR uses while the client focuses on upsetting memories from the past. He said, "Oh, you blank out the emotions around the issue." I thought, "How the heck does he know that?" I was shocked. Then he asked me to come to his home that night and try it with him. I was shocked again.

I went to his home and asked if he had an issue that he would like to focus on when we did the technique. He said he did and explained what it was. Everyone goes through things in life that overwhelm them, so I was not that surprised that he could come up with a suitable topic to address. It was a big issue, though. Assuming it would take more than one session, I was already mentally trying to figure out when I could come back and meet with him a few more times to finish the work.

We went through the preliminary processes and then started the Desensitization Phase, the part that gets rid of the bad feelings. EMDR usually works quickly to remove those feelings. Often if the issue is a single incident the bad feelings might be gone in one or two sessions that are an hour and a half in length. In this case they were gone in about five minutes. I was confused. I thought maybe his emotions just muted for a while and would resurface if we kept doing the processing, so I kept going for a while. After about ten more minutes I had to concede that the Desensitization Phase was finished. The Positive Installation Phase and the Body Scan had finished automatically as well. We discussed the experience and Master Chia had many positive things to say about it. I walked away from that experience feeling very happy but confused.

The next day at lunch Master Chia called me over to his table and said, "You know, that EMDR works but the emotions are still in the organs." At first I thought that we had somehow missed something in the Body Scan. Then he started to explain how EMDR works from an energy perspective and how it actually validates what Taoist masters have been saying and teaching for millennia, especially the part about eye movement.

However, as Einstein coined it in his famous equation $E=MC^2$, energy cannot be created or destroyed. It can only be transformed. EMDR removes the connection between the mind and the memory, but the emotion around that issue is not gone. It is still in the internal organs. Think of it like a computer where the brain is the hardware, the organs are the software, and there are links to each file. EMDR destroys the link but leaves the energy in the organs. The file name has been messed up. The energetic residue of that issue does not know where to go now. It could go anywhere. Energy that has not been transformed can come back to the person through a new route. The energy in the organs still needs to be transformed and grounded to the earth so it will not come back to the person.

As Master Chia and I continued our discussions, we both thought that the Universal Healing Tao Chi Kung system could help to explain, improve, and transform the EMDR technique into something that people could reliably and effectively use to heal themselves. In order to understand how these benefits could arise from their combination, it is important to have some understanding of Taoism, chi, and Chi Kung.

Taoism

Taoism is an ancient Chinese philosophy that focuses on learning how to live in harmony with nature. Lao Tzu is given credit for developing Taoism and putting its teachings in writing in the Tao Te Ching. Taoist practices involve developing our awareness of the energies in and around us and learning how best to respond to them. Balance is emphasized in Taoist teachings, which can be seen in these two selections from the Tao Te Ching (translated by Stephen Mitchell):

> *The Tao doesn't take sides;*
> *it gives birth to both good and evil.*
> *The Master doesn't take sides;*
> *she welcomes both saints and sinners.*
>
> *The Tao is like a bellows;*
> *it is empty yet infinitely capable.*
> *The more you use it, the more it produces;*
> *the more you talk of it, the less you understand.*

Relaxation and letting go are also important concepts to embrace in Taoism. As the ancient system of Taoism evolved over thousands of years, it cultivated many aspects of health and healing, such as acupuncture, Tai Chi, Feng Shui (the art of placement in the home or office to create harmonious energy flow), the I Ching (a method of tapping into universal energy for guidance about how to approach future events), Chinese astrology, and Chi Kung.

Chi and Chi Kung

Chi (pronounced "chee") is the energy around and within us. Different cultures and systems have named it differently, but there seems to be widespread agreement that chi exists. Western science, for example, refers to the bioelectromagnetic energy of the body. In our bodies, chi travels on all levels and through all types of tissues. Blood follows where the chi goes. There are different types of chi in our bodies, on our planet, and in the universe.

Chi Kung refers to the process of learning how to master those energies, to manage, heal, strengthen, and balance health on all levels so that we can more easily create inner harmony and interact harmoniously with the world around us. It helps us to have a clearer sense of our best options for responding to our circumstances in ways that do not disrupt harmony. When people practice Chi Kung they experience a natural high. Chi is relaxed energy, so they feel calm and centered, but they also feel energetic enough to respond to the situations of the day. People who practice Chi Kung learn how to slow down, relax, concentrate, store energy, and conduct themselves in ways that do not waste their energy or burn it too quickly.

Like many aboriginal and ancient cultures, Chi Kung has focused on how to live in harmony with nature and to learn from it. Many Chi Kung practices were developed from watching how children, animals, and trees respond to changing conditions. Working on the body in this way allows people to bypass some of their resistance to change. For example, thinking about relaxation might bring up thoughts of why now is not a good time to relax, but proper breathing often brings about a state of relaxation without any objections or resistance.

The focus on symptoms in Western medicine has resulted in one person often receiving treatment from many different specialists, each with his or her own perspective (often conflicting), and many treatments for a single person, each with their own set of side effects. In contrast, the perspective offered by Chi Kung and all the practices of the Universal Tao system is one that recognizes the body-mind as a single integrated system.

SHARING OUR DISCOVERIES

From the discussions that followed my first interchange with Master Chia about EMDR, we mutually realized that the combination of EMDR with the Universal Healing Tao system of Chi Kung principles and practices provided the raw material to develop a new method that can be used to teach people how to heal themselves. Over the years we have independently experimented with combining elements of EMDR with Chi Kung and have shared our experiences and discoveries at various points along the way. The practice of what we refer to as Taoist Emotional Recycling has been refined to the point where it now makes sense to share it with everyone and provide a new and powerful way to heal.

Perhaps you have wondered, "How can we stray from a healthy and happy path?" and "How can we tell that we have strayed from it?" The material presented in the first five chapters covers how external influences can lead us to become confused about how to live in harmony with the world. These chapters make it clear that we often think and operate in ways that confuse us further, leading to ineffective and complicated "solutions," as well as to conditions like depression, anxiety, and trauma.

This book was written to shed light on the energetic connections between mood disturbances like depression and anxiety with trauma and addictions, and to show how this new energetic method can dissolve and transform those connections. Starting with chapter 6 you will learn how insights from Taoism, the Universal Healing Tao, and EMDR can be used to create a simple and yet powerful practice that can overturn these dynamics and thus help you to heal yourself and others on all levels.

The practice is consistent with the principles of the Universal Healing Tao system and with the tenets of Taoism, which help to clarify how and why the method works—holistically, with the whole mind-body system. Quotes from the Tao Te Ching are sprinkled in relevant sections throughout the book. Notice your reactions to the ideas that are presented. They may give you some ideas about how you have been unknowingly influenced in ways that have moved you from your basic nature and true purpose.

In order to highlight the factors that seem important, terms like "people" and "modern society" are used to refer to the general tendencies of some groups, not to suggest that every person in the world operates in the same way. The illustrations often purposefully offer oversimplified or exaggerated situations to make a specific point. Please receive them with the lightness in which they are offered.

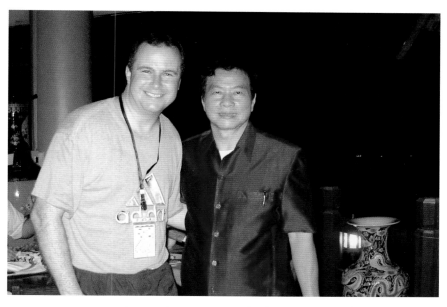

Doug Hilton and Master Mantak Chia at Tao Garden
during Tao Congress in 2010

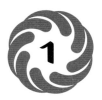

Searching for Meaning and Health in the Modern World

We all seem to be searching for similar things: inner peace, emotional control, ways to shut off unwanted thoughts, physical health and vitality, an understanding of the principles upon which life operates, and an understanding of how best to respond to life as it presents us with changes and challenges. Each of us searches at our own pace and in our own way for answers. In our modern world there are so many options to explore. One person may turn to religion for answers, another may embrace a particular branch of science, and another may turn to alternative or complementary health practices. Each of these has merit, of course, but may not provide a complete enough explanation and experience to satisfy the individual seeker. It is a common experience that even when people find a belief system that is satisfying, and when they know what they should do, think, or feel, they do not know how to put those intentions into action. Addictive quick fixes can seem simpler and more reliable than the work that it takes to find or make our own magic in life, but they do not produce the same kind of lasting satisfaction that the journey to genuine happiness can bring.

LOSING OUR WAY

In general, we all know that we are supposed to "do the right thing," but how do you know what that is in each given situation? During times of confusion and struggle, friends and relatives will tell us to "be strong," "don't give up without a fight," and "listen to your gut," but at other times they will tell us to "take the good with the bad," "let it go," and "use your head." When are we supposed to "turn the other cheek" and when are we supposed to "stick to our guns"? If we do not have a foundation of knowledge and practice to help us know how and when to do what, even well-meaning advice can be very confusing. How are we supposed to develop self-discipline if we do not know how our various mental, emotional, and physical systems work or how they are connected to and affected by our environment?

Without knowing how to sort out what our approach should be, most of us react out of fear and rely solely on our willpower and logic to get us through life. The trouble, of course, is that life does not always conform to our will or our personal ideas of how things should be. When we overuse our willpower to control things, we tend to get into power struggles with our friends, bosses, family, spouses, and coworkers. Anger, frustration, fear, worry, and resentment can build as we discover time and again that—no matter how clear we are in our minds about

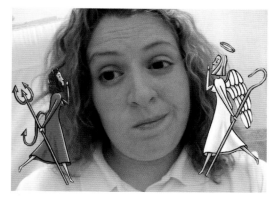

Fig. 1.1. Contradictory messages create confusion.

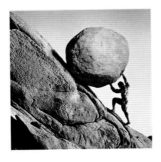

Fig. 1.2. Trying to control the uncontrollable can feel like you are trying to push a large boulder up a hill.

what should happen in life—we will not always get our way. We can even become overwhelmed when our experiences are too far from our beliefs about the world or ourselves. Overwhelming feelings can lead to anxiety and depression.

Mass media reinforces the idea of turning to some external source to feel better. The reminders and encouragement are all around us—in magazines, in books, on television, on billboards, and on the web. The message might be encouraging you to do something unhealthy like drink alcohol, do drugs, smoke cigarettes, eat excessively, or gamble. Or it might be encouraging you to do something healthy such as reading a book,

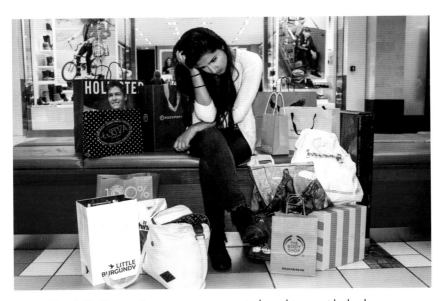

Fig. 1.3. Our society encourages us to buy things with the hope that those things will make us happy.

watching a funny movie, visiting with friends, or joining a meditation class. Even when we can access those healthy external sources, striving for more and better external things to make us feel better only provides temporary relief from our stress and confusion. Other messages reinforce the idea that the accumulation of stuff will make us happy, but there is no guarantee that we will always have the money to buy those things.

Another aspect of our modern society that unwittingly contributes to the need for people to resort to external solutions for their problems is our emphasis on fairness. Fairness is woven into our culture through the mass media. We all like hearing stories about good triumphing over evil. Unfortunately the combination of encouraging people to control their environments and their destinies through willpower with the idea that fairness is expected and desirable in life is a recipe for failure, disillusionment, and feeling overwhelmed.

Sometimes people end up doing something unhealthy like alcohol, drugs, or gambling to cope with those overwhelmed feelings. Some people end up dependent on some addictive substance or activity. Addiction and trauma are key and pervasive factors in most of the crimes and injustices that we perpetrate against each other. Most of us have probably asked at one time or another, "What is wrong with people?" and "Why can't we just get along?" We wonder why there is so much war, deceit, and thievery over money, objects, and land. However, those behaviors could be viewed as by-products of a world that supports the accumulation of things as the solution to our problems.

Many of our formal efforts to change such patterns have been to create specialized services and expert positions to tackle each part of the problem. We have put a lot of time, energy, and money into dividing problems up into subcategories, coming up with names for those subcategories, and creating policies, laws, services, training programs, and supporting paperwork to document our progress in addressing the issues. We create procedures and positions for evaluation of that progress. We restructure organizations based on these evaluations. Soon we will need to have experts to tell us which experts to access to get help

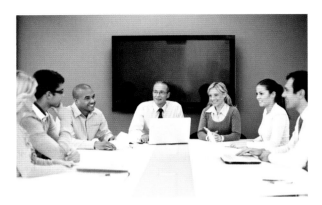

Fig. 1.4. Logic and willpower seem useful on the surface, but sometimes they can lead us to solutions that create more problems and complexity.

for our problems. But is this approach really giving us the results we want? It does not seem like it. The wars on crime, drugs, terror, and poverty have not been won. Our strategies to deal with the symptoms are based on the same source beliefs of logic and willpower that created those problems in the first place.

In short, we live in a world that seems dominated by the idea of striving to soothe our suffering and yet our suffering is a result of that same striving. This can lead to unhealthy beliefs and habits that are woven so tightly into our individual beliefs and habits that we do not notice or stop to question them.

LIVING IN A QUICK-FIX SOCIETY

Media bombards us regularly with the latest and quickest ways to help us feel better, save time, and reach our goals. Quick fixes are celebrated; they seem so appealing and meet many needs at once. For example, people smoke cigarettes to relax, to be social, to feel cool or sophisticated, and to get more energy. A fix feels convenient and efficient. It is no surprise that people turn to more drastic and dangerous quick fixes when the ones that they usually use are not working or if they do not have healthier alternatives. Using quick fixes as a lifestyle creates a paradoxical pattern. People end up trying to use quick fixes to relax. However, if that strategy does not work, they find themselves unable to relax. Then they have a tendency to try more dangerous quick fixes

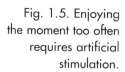

Fig. 1.5. Enjoying the moment too often requires artificial stimulation.

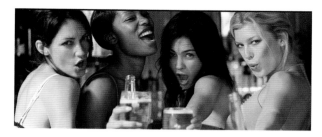

so that they can relax. Cycles like this could be avoided if they learned how to do the opposite—relax first and then go fix whatever remains to be addressed after that.

PARENTS CANNOT COMPLETELY COUNTERBALANCE THE INFLUENCE OF SOCIETY

Parents are often held responsible for how their children fare emotionally and financially in life. However, how can parents offer enough guidance and influence to offset the influence of the various media that are encouraging children to strive in life and to measure their worth by how many things they can purchase, especially considering that parents are influenced in similar ways? Without an understanding of how societal expectations have affected their parents' happiness, it is easy for

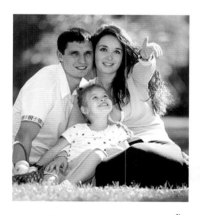
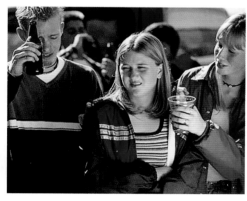

Fig. 1.6. Our parents influence how we approach life a great deal, but society influences us as well.

children to blame their parents. Ironically, carrying around resentments uses up a lot of energy and weakens people, thereby making them even more susceptible to becoming overwhelmed or depressed as they deal with the challenges in their lives.

RACING TO FILL
YOUR LIFE CAN LEAVE
YOU FEELING EMPTY INSIDE

Living in a Competitive Society

Our world runs on money. Some people have more than others. We cannot have the things we want without money, so we compete for money, power, and status in the hope that we will then have those things one day. Some people will win those competitions, while others will lose. We will all lose at times. We notice when that happens and tend to feel down, at least for a while. We tend to put pressure on ourselves to do more and better so we can get the money and things we want. That can create stress and anxiety.

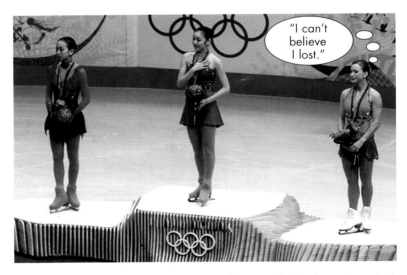

Fig. 1.7. Trying to win as a lifestyle will eventually lead people to feel disappointed and resentful.

Too Much Attachment, Not Enough Detachment

In our consumerist culture we are bombarded on a daily basis with messages from media of all kinds that we need to buy and achieve things to be a success. We are encouraged to "fight for what is ours." We end up clinging to our belongings as a result. Such attachment increases the likelihood that we will cling to other things in our lives as well, such as people, emotions, and our point of view. Detachment can seem unnecessary or undesirable to people who operate in this way. However, it is inevitable that we will lose things. We will not always get what we want. So if we have not learned to detach or to appreciate the value of detachment, we run a higher risk of becoming overwhelmed when life does not provide us with the things that we want or think we should have. A common goal that is expressed in addiction recovery is to "detach with love." Although that sounds appealing, many people do not know how to put it into action. It is difficult to let go of attachments if most of our lifestyle involves striving and grasping.

In chapter 9 of the Tao Te Ching, Lao Tzu shows us another way:

> *Hanging on to it will cause overflow; better to*
> *let go.*
> *Forced consent does not endure.*
> *Filling the house with gold and jade will not*
> *bring safety.*

Fig. 1.8. Striving and grasping in life will eventually lead to unhappiness if a person does not also know how to detach and let go when striving for more becomes pointless.

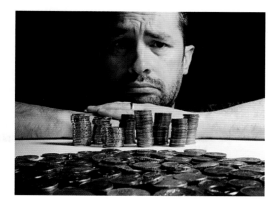

*Riches and royalty result in pride; they bring
about their own punishment.
When the work is done, the body withdraws.
This is the Tao of heaven.*

Note: This and all subsequent selections quoted from the Tao Te Ching are from *Secret Teachings of the Tao Te Ching,* by Mantak Chia and Tao Huang.

Lack of Knowledge of the Natural Process of Change

As a result of linear thinking, extreme living, and moving too fast, many people tend to develop expectations of themselves and of life that are unreasonable. They expect change to happen quickly and easily, even if they are trying to change a problem that has affected many areas of their lives for years. There is a tendency to expect change to happen in

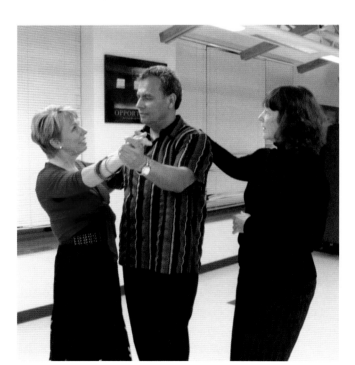

Fig. 1.9. Relax and enjoy the process.

a linear way, with no ups and downs along the way. Such people often focus too much on the outcome instead of the process and therefore do not give themselves credit for any progress that they make until they achieve their goals. That is called perfectionism. Perfectionists treat mistakes as reflections of character flaws instead of merely opportunities for learning and growth. People who do not understand the natural process of change also develop faulty thinking about how much control they have or should have over the events in their lives. What is needed is to relax and enjoy the process, including the natural ups and downs that come with learning something new.

All of these misperceptions of the natural process of change set people up for disappointment and increase the risk that they will end up feeling overwhelmed by life. Obsessing and ruminating are often the coping strategies of people who are overwhelmed in this way. They are trying to find a solution, but the linear thinking that they are using to solve it puts them in a loop with no solution. Meanwhile the toxic emotional energy is piling up inside of them as they struggle to sort it out. Fear created by a lack of knowledge or faith in the natural order of things can increase the likelihood that they will turn to activities and substances that will actually create more chaos and confusion in their lives.

Devaluing and Not Understanding the Need to Let Go

In a world that emphasizes the accumulation of goods to measure success and worth in life, it is natural for us to adopt an approach that supports the goal. We tend to try to go straight toward our goals and view any obstacles in our path as problems or threats. Any time we cannot continue to go forward toward them is viewed as a personal failure. We start thinking that shame and guilt are necessary to spur us on to learn our lessons and do better next time. However, shame and guilt undermine our confidence and increase the chances that we will continue to create unsuccessful results. We need to understand that we all grow and

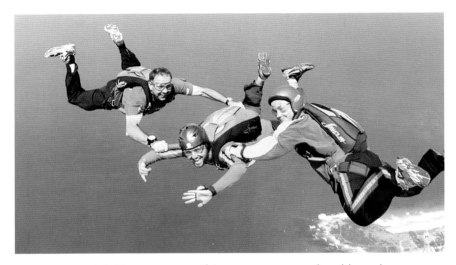

Fig. 1.10. There are some things we may never be able to do.

learn at our own pace, with ups and downs along the way. We all have strengths and challenges. There are some things we may never be able to do. Letting go has to do with acceptance of the reality of the situation and of our own limits of control over ourselves and a situation; it has nothing to do with being lazy or weak.

Not Focusing Enough on the Present

Striving for material success naturally encourages focusing on the future. Too much focus on the future can create worry, which reduces our enjoyment of the present moment. Not focusing on the present limits our concentration on and control of the present. A lack of focus on the present will tend to produce less success in meeting our goals. Then we tend to feel bad about our limited success, which draws our attention back to the past. Not focusing on the present leaves people with bad feelings.

An Attitude That Lacks Gratitude

Consumerism without a spiritual base to keep it in perspective can leave us vulnerable to the sophisticated methods of advertising that suggest

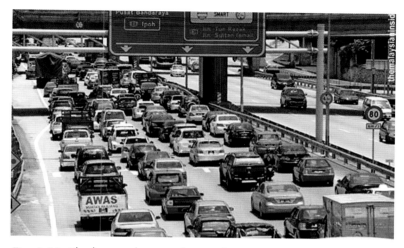

Fig. 1.11. The latest advances do not always create greater happiness.

that unless we buy all the latest products on the market we cannot be happy. Then we inevitably discover that the enjoyment from owning those products is short-lived. Following that type of lifestyle limits how much enjoyment we can take from what we already have, especially those aspects of our lives that are not material possessions.

SUCCESSFUL VS. UNSUCCESSFUL STRATEGIES

Confusing Assertiveness with Aggression

In keeping with our societal approach that involves grasping, striving, and collecting, we often redefine assertiveness to mean making people do what we want rather than just letting people know what we want or need. This puts us out of balance in terms of our beliefs about our personal power. That can lead us to operate as if we should be able to get whatever we want and to feel guilt and shame if we don't. We also tend to feel anger, frustration, and resentment toward the people and situations that do not bow to our will. Habitually trying to get our way through coercion and manipulation often leads to more frustration because other people always have the option to say "no."

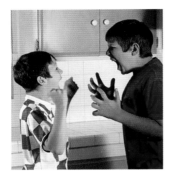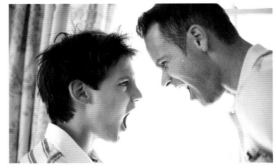

Fig. 1.12. Unbalanced beliefs about personal power can lead
to anger, frustration, and resentment toward the people and
situations that do not bow to our will.

Overusing Willpower

Some aspects of our lives can be influenced by our effort while others
are beyond our control. One general way of making the distinction is
that we have control over ourselves but not much control over others. If
someone else is determined to not do what we want then our control is
very limited. Willpower cannot overcome physical limits or the practical realities of a situation.

If people are living a materialistic lifestyle, admitting that they cannot
always get what they want may not seem like a very appealing thought. As
a result people tend to ignore the reality of the limits of their influence
and overuse their willpower in aggressive and manipulative ways.

Accidentally Setting Off Our Defense Systems

Without knowing another way to approach bad habits, we often use
our upper brains to try to win the battle between our conscious and
unconscious minds. However, when we try to tell ourselves to do something while we have some reservations on a deeper level, we accidentally
activate our defense systems to keep us from acting on our conscious
desires.

Imagine someone who is afraid of heights telling himself or herself
to look over the edge of a skyscraper. The more he or she tries to do

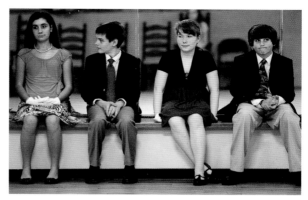

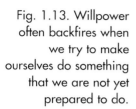

Fig. 1.13. Willpower often backfires when we try to make ourselves do something that we are not yet prepared to do.

it, the more the reasons not to look would come to mind. The person might think something like "Are you crazy? I'm really scared!" In many cases working with the body works better because those same defense systems do not come up as easily. The Universal Healing Tao and the Tao Te Ching, upon which it is based, portray a healthier approach that goes "beyond the power of will":

> *The ancient sages of Tao are subtle and mysteriously*
> *penetrating.*
> *Their depth is beyond the power of will.*
> *Because it is beyond the power of will,*
> *The most we can do is describe it:*
> *Thus, full of care, as one crossing the wintry stream,*
> *Attentive, as one cautious of the total environment,*
> *Reserved, as one who is a guest,*
> *Spread open, as when confronting a marsh,*
> *Simple, like uncarved wood, opaque, like mud,*
> *Magnificent, like a valley.*
> *From within the murky comes the stillness.*
> *The feminine enlivens with her milk.*
> *Keeping such a Tao, excess is undesirable.*
> *Desiring no excess, work is completed without*
> *exhaustion.*

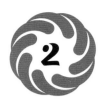

Going to Extremes Can Keep You Off Balance

The waterways of planet Earth offer us a helpful way to think about the energy systems in our body: they are like a system of waterways of various shapes and sizes, like oceans, rivers, lakes, and streams. Think about what happens to those waterways as you learn about each of the factors that follow.

THE SEARCH FOR HAPPINESS CAN LEAD TO AN UNHEALTHY AND EXTREME LIFESTYLE

In our hectic modern world, where we are scrambling to make enough money to buy the next invention that is supposed to make our lives enjoyable or save time, we can easily become so stressed that we are overwhelmed.

Extreme behavior and extreme desire are celebrated in many aspects of modern society. Common phrases like "Go big or go home" and "Whoever dies with the most toys wins" are examples of that sentiment.

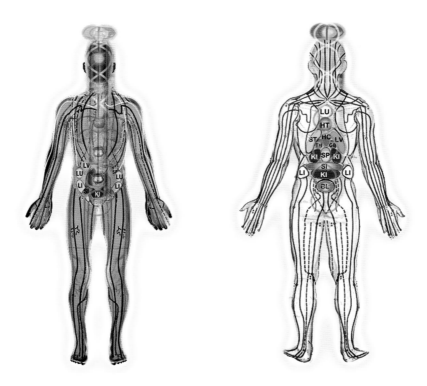

Fig. 2.1. The energetic systems in the human body are like rivers, lakes, streams, and oceans.

Such ideas encourage people to put more emphasis on external results than internal peace and to strive for a life that is out of balance. Sometimes it even goes so far as to suggest that having external results will create internal peace. However, we all know that is not a guarantee and "more" and "bigger" are not always better. In fact, the type of striving, grasping, and competing that occurs when people believe that that is their only or best option for happiness often creates too much stress and robs them of their natural enjoyment of life.

Moving Too Fast

When we get into difficult situations many of us will go faster to try to hurry up and sort things out before the situation becomes worse.

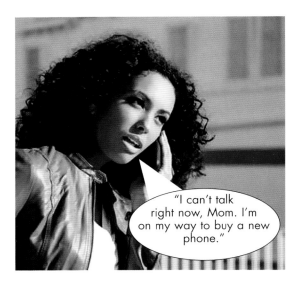

Fig. 2.2. We rely too much on technology, "more," and "faster" to make our lives better.

"I can't talk right now, Mom. I'm on my way to buy a new phone."

Unfortunately that increases the chance that we will end up feeling overwhelmed, not necessarily because the situation is getting worse but just because it is more stressful to try to manage a difficult situation by going faster than it is by slowing down. A saying that might help you to remember not to fall into the trap of going faster is "Under stress, we regress." When we are stressed we tend to use the responses that are most familiar to us. We do not usually want to try something new at those times because that might be even more stressful. Our old, familiar ways of handling things tend to be ones that we learned earlier in life when we had less knowledge and experience, so creating more stress for ourselves by moving too quickly usually does not help the situation.

State-Dependent Learning

Another concept that might help us to understand why moving more slowly is actually better when we are dealing with difficult situations is State-Dependent Learning. We tend to remember the things that we learn when we are in the same state that we were in when we first learned those lessons. If most of your best coping strategies were learned when you were in a calm state, you will be more likely to remember them when you are in a calm state. We usually learn things at work or

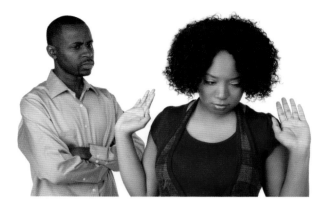

Fig. 2.3. State-Dependent Learning refers to the tendency of people to forget what they know when they are in a different state than they were when they first gained that knowledge.

in school when we are calm. If we later develop a frantic or chaotic life-style it will be more difficult to access the information that we need to function at our best in the world, including the awareness of how much more effective we are when we are calm.

If you get too stressed you may not be able to access your best store of information and strategies. Couples are often baffled by this dynamic when they get into arguments. In the heat of an argument they tend to respond in ways that are uncharacteristic of them and even in ways that cross lines that they promised themselves that they would never cross.

Too Much Heat

Moving too fast, thinking too much, pushing ourselves to get the latest gadgets and conveniences and living an extreme lifestyle create friction and heat in the body. Heat rises. Stressed people end up with too much heat in their heads. Then they cannot think clearly or sleep soundly. Having too much heat can contribute to what we call "burnout." Intuitively we seem to know this is true. Notice that we sometimes refer to our brain as being "fried" when we are too stressed and cannot think clearly.

Too much heat in the top half of the body can make it difficult for us to think clearly or to calm down. Notice that we say "calm down." No one says "calm up." We all seem to be aware on some level that relaxation and cooling off are connected concepts. When we cannot sleep properly or think clearly we tend to make poor decisions and our performance

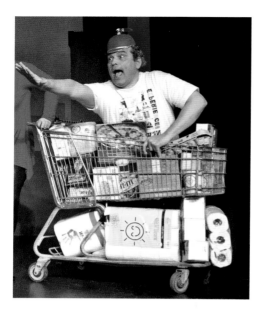

Fig. 2.4. A frantic pace creates too much heat, which negatively affects our ability to be effective.

is hindered, which brings undesirable consequences, which in turn puts more stress on us to fix the problems that have developed as a result of our poor decisions and performance. Worrying about and trying to fix the new problems can create more heat and friction. It is a vicious cycle. That kind of heat can also contribute to hyperactivity or make it worse.

Too Much Tension

Many people view relaxation as something to mostly be addressed on holidays and vacations. Not only does that put a lot of pressure on those events to provide all the stress reduction that a person needs, but it also makes relaxation an event rather than an ongoing process. With phrases like "no pain, no gain," "work before play," "man up," and "working for the weekend," we seem to have embraced a lifestyle that has relegated the restorative aspect of life to a low priority, in which it is only allowed after we have accomplished whatever our goals are. When we get tense, though, we tend to perform less effectively, so such an approach greatly increases the likelihood that we will become depressed, stressed, and overwhelmed.

In Taoist terms, many people live a lifestyle that is out of balance in that it puts too much emphasis on the yang (aggressive, active) aspect of life and not enough on the yin (restorative, receiving) aspect. Think of it as a bank account. If you withdraw more than you have, you will be in trouble, which Lao Tzu makes clear in chapter 26 of the Tao Te Ching.

> *The heavy is the root of the light.*
> *Tranquility is the master of the restless.*
> *Thus, the noble person will travel all day without*
>   *leaving his seat.*
> *Though the center of the highest authority,*
> *And surrounded by luxury,*
> *He remains clear-minded.*
> *How could the king of myriad chariots treat his*
>   *body with less care than he gives the country?*
> *Being careless loses the foundation.*
> *Being restless loses mastery.*

Too Tight

A lot of emphasis is put on having a tight body, especially in the abdominal area. Being thin and tight is fine, and contracting your muscles is necessary during exercise, but if people hold their bodies tight all the time then they will end up feeling tired and stressed. The energy channels in your body are like tiny garden hoses. If you kink the hoses, the flow will be impeded.

Our internal organs are responsible for processing our food and liquids. They need to be relaxed and able to move freely so they can do their work. Ironically, if people hold their abdomens too tight their food will take longer to go through the digestive process. That makes it more likely that their food will end up being stored as fat. People whose bodies are routinely too tight will perform less effectively in the rest of their daily activities and feel slow and irritable as they struggle to overcome their energetic constraints. This can lead to feeling depressed, anxious, and even overwhelmed.

When people are born, they are soft and gentle.
When they die, they are stiff and callous.
When myriad things, grasses, and trees, are born,
   they are soft and tender.
When they die, they are withered.
So stiffness and callousness are the company of death.
Softness and suppleness are the company of life.
The powerful army will not win.
A stiff tree will break.
So stiffness and power stay below.
Softness and suppleness stay above.

(TAO TE CHING, CHAPTER 78)

Lack of Body Awareness

Despite how important our bodies are to us and how much their condition can affect our enjoyment of life, many of us still do not know our bodies very well. If you asked a room full of people to locate their spleen, for example, many people would not be able to. Not being knowledgeable about or aware of our bodies puts us in a position where we do not know how to take the best care of ourselves, especially in preventive ways.

LIVING TOO SENSUALLY

We can also become overwhelmed if we focus too much on the material world that we sense with our eyes, ears, nose, mouth, and tongue, without giving enough attention to the spiritual and energetic side of life that underlies it. Striving and competing can become a lifestyle. The quest for money, possessions, conquests, status, and power can leave us feeling unfulfilled. We all lose, fail, make mistakes, and get old. The relentless chase for material success can lead to premature aging and heart attacks. We can become very tired and unhappy from chasing after things that we hope will make us happy. A life without mean-

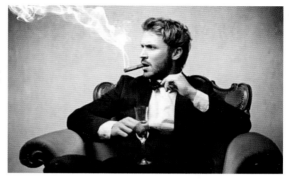

Fig. 2.5. "I'm bored.
Now what?"

ing beyond what can be experienced through the senses will eventually become unfulfilling, as Lao Tzu makes clear in chapter 12 of the Tao Te Ching:

> *Five colors blind the eyes.*
> *Racing and hunting madden the heart.*
> *Pursuing what is rare makes action deceitful.*
> *Five flavors dull the palate. Five tones deafen the ears.*
> *So the sage's method is for the belly not the eyes.*
> *He abandons the latter and chooses the former.*

Avoiding too much emphasis on pleasing our senses and remembering that they are only our filters for reality rather than reality itself can help us to not get too caught up in power struggles with the people and situations in our lives. Creating a beautiful and expansive environment inside ourselves is far more obtainable than trying to buy one.

Focusing outward on external bright and colorful, loud, tasty, and fragrant things to make us happy can in fact make us tired and unhappy. Using our senses too much does not let them rest properly. We expend energy trying to experience those sensory delights and our energy tends to crash afterward. Extreme amounts of sensory stimulation can seem exhilarating at the time, but they drain us later. Being exposed too often to extreme amounts of stimulation can dull our senses to the

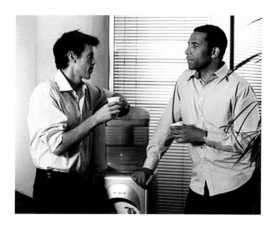

Fig. 2.6. "I finally met a woman who is stable, sane, kind, considerate, and fun. The only problem is she's so boring."

extraordinary wonders of everyday life and create a tendency toward dependencies on substances and exciting activities. This creates a downward spiral of depression, using stimulation to medicate it, and more of a crash after the medicating wears off. Flooding your senses on a regular basis will make it difficult to appreciate the peace of everyday moments.

Adaptation Taken Too Far

Human beings are built to adapt to the circumstances around them. As we move further and further from our natural state to respond to the demands of daily life, the stress, frustration, and overstimulation of that lifestyle eventually starts to feel normal. A slower, less extreme lifestyle starts to seem boring. We become used to a rollercoaster ride of dramatic highs and lows. That ride is very wearing on our internal systems. Eventually people start to feel tired from it and need more extreme highs to restore their energy temporarily. Meanwhile toxins accumulate as they push themselves beyond their natural limits.

GOING AGAINST OUR BASIC NATURE

In order to keep up with the hectic pace and expectations of modern life, we often end up living in ways that our bodies would not naturally require. We eat and drink quickly at meals, wake up earlier than our bodies seem to want, and use stimulants like caffeine, cigarettes, and alcohol to keep us going even after our bodies are exhausted. As a result we are more vulnerable than ever to feeling burned out, depressed, anxious, or overwhelmed.

Emptying More Than Filling

When we get stressed our bodies naturally prepare us to run away or fight. It is referred to as the "fight-or-flight" response. At those times our kidneys contract and pull tight like a muscle and the diaphragm muscle pulls tight all the way across the bottom of the ribcage in the front of the body. That makes it difficult to breathe fully. The top of the abdominal cavity is pulled tight so there is not much room for air to get in. Even after the threat is over, the body tends to stay on a type of "yellow alert" with shallow breathing. It can stay that way for weeks, months, or even years. In the meantime our bodies are not being flushed out properly and so toxins and tension build in the body.

Somehow many of us have taken some good notions like "Treat others the way you would like to be treated" and "It's better to give

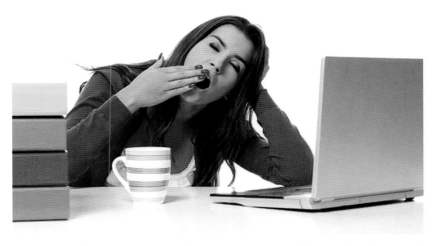

Fig. 2.7. "The boss can't wait till tomorrow. Guess I'll be working late again tonight." People who push themselves too hard will eventually turn to stimulants to help themselves keep going.

than to receive" to extremes, to the point where they are now taken to mean that to receive from others or take care of yourself is selfish. But people pleasing can create dependency. It wears out the person who is doing the pleasing and robs the receiver of learning how to manage on his or her own. Too much self-sacrifice ultimately leads people to burn themselves out physically, emotionally, mentally, and spiritually. If that continues for long enough the person will not be able to help anyone else either. To combat this, 12-step programs often refer to the need for a "self first" approach rather than a selfish one.

Removing Ourselves from Nature Leads to Unnatural Habits

Modern technological life has helped to protect us from the harsh aspects of nature like storms and cold, but it has also helped us to disconnect from nature in general. Other than weekend getaways and holidays, we tend to remain away from natural scenes. Now we pay large amounts of money and work hard so that we can get away from the city life that was supposed to help us get away from nature. When we get back to nature we are reminded of what peace feels like and how to move more in sync with the flow of life. When we are away from it we forget and sometimes end up turning to stimulants to help us move faster than the cycles of life so we can stay ahead of them. Unfortu-

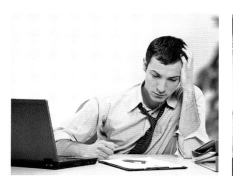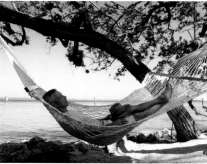

Fig. 2.8. A balanced and happy life involves regularly taking breaks from the hectic and complicated aspects of our lives.

nately that often leads to impatience, frustration, and careless errors, which compounds our desire to "get away."

Too Tired to Grow and Flow

Pushing ourselves beyond our natural limits in pursuit of what we have been led to believe will give us happiness creates consequences that can leave us feeling old before our time. We may feel tired and then, even if we realize that our lifestyle needs to change, we may not have the reserve energy to make the changes that are needed.

Defining success by external results also affects our priorities. Consciously or not, if we are busy striving for more money, status, property, and fame, we tend to not believe that we have time or energy to look after our bodies or emotions. Then, if we reach for "quick fixes" like alcohol, drugs, and gambling when times are tough, our energetic pathways become blocked with toxins and filled with weak and stagnant energy, which makes it even more difficult for us to achieve our goals.

IMMATERIAL BECOMES MATERIAL

Many people do not know about or pay enough attention to the toxins that are piling up inside of them. Toxins can come to us through the air we breathe, the food we eat, the things we drink, our emotions, and the emotions of others. They all take up energetic space inside us. The toxins clog our meridians, the energetic pathways of the body. That leads us to feel more and more stuck and distressed on a physical, emotional, mental, and spiritual level. We develop various chronic conditions when this happens. Then we feel weighted down by life and have a sense that it would take very little to push us past the point of what we can take. We end up being more fearful and irritable as a result and, ironically, that makes us even more likely to build up emotional toxins inside. It becomes a vicious cycle.

Our ability to think clearly and sharply is affected, too. On some

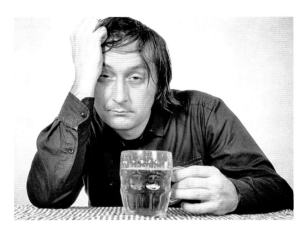

Fig. 2.9. Extreme living leads to toxic build-up. Toxic build-up leads to poorer performance and results, and often to self-medication in an attempt to cope with bad feelings.

level we all seem to know this. When we refer to people who are not thinking properly we often use terms like "thick" and "dense." If people do not understand the connection between toxins and bad feelings they are more likely to turn to something extreme, and possibly addictive, to make themselves feel better, which will lead to even more toxins developing in their systems.

Lacking Self-Discipline Training

How do we learn to relax, concentrate, and follow through on our ideas? It is rare for us to be simply born with those abilities. If we are not trained in how to do these things, or, even worse, are shown poor examples of self-discipline as we grow up, we are more likely to resort

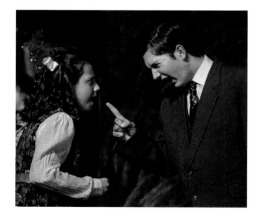

Fig. 2.10. "Calm down, would you?? What is wrong with you??" People who have not learned self-discipline often try to control the people and situations around them instead.

to quick fixes. If we cannot control ourselves we will try to control the people and things around us. However, not only is control of external events not possible, but often people will "dig their heels in" and do the opposite of what we want. This is a formula for eventual hurt feelings that will pile up inside of us over time.

TOO MUCH STIMULATION CAN BE A REAL DOWNER

Modern society is strewn with stimulants. People use caffeine, nicotine, methamphetamine, gambling, sex, shopping, cocaine, and a variety of prescriptions to help them maintain a hectic lifestyle. Of course, what goes up must come down. The crash from stimulants after their effects wear off leaves people feeling worse than before they took them. The desired effects of stimulants also tend to become less noticeable with

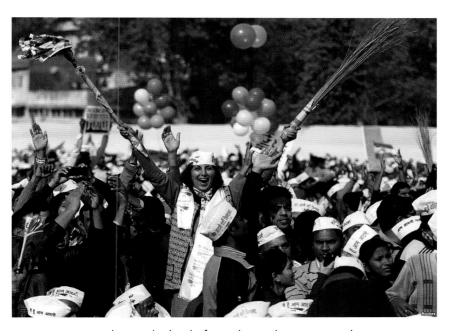

Fig. 2.11. We adapt to the level of stimulation that we use to keep us going. Over time we hardly notice the effects of the stimulants, so we need more. We can easily lose track of how much our daily lives are fueled by stimulants.

continued use, to the point where people often eventually do not feel them at all. This creates another vicious downward spiral as people chase a feeling that slips further away from them.

Speedy Media

In our modern world we have various kinds of media images and information bombarding us. The information is fed to us in quick and colorful ways so we will be able to focus on the whole message without getting bored or distracted. As a result many of us end up with poorly developed powers of concentration. When we need to concentrate it will be difficult, which will lead to poorer results on various tasks, which increases the risk that we will become depressed, stressed, overwhelmed. Getting things quickly comes at a price. We lose the ability to wait and to focus on what we want.

Lack of Knowledge of How to Manage Our Sexual Energy

Sex sells. Everyone knows it. As a result, a lot of the mass media uses sexual stimulation to sell products and promote the ideas that keep our materialistic culture going. Sex is one of our basic drives. It is our best energy, the one that can produce life. Yet most of us do not know how to regulate our sexual energy or how to share that energy with the rest of our systems in beneficial ways. For more information about how to accomplish those things, check out one of the books on that subject by Master Mantak Chia in the bibliography. Without knowledge of how to regulate their sexual energy people are vulnerable to mass media campaigns that pair the promise of sexual stimulation and satisfaction with various products that they do not really need to be happy.

Lack of Knowledge of the Dopamine Connection

Dopamine is a naturally-occurring neurotransmitter in the brain that is released when we feel stimulated. It helps to regulate our moods. However, many people do not know that overindulging in certain activities will lead to more dopamine being released than we need. Excessive eating, gambling, sex, interpersonal drama, and shopping are examples of activities that can affect the dopamine levels in the brain. Eventually the body will crave more of that good feeling. If people are not aware of that connection, they may think that there is no harm in overindulging and could end up with a dependency or an addiction. In addition, due to that lack of knowledge, they will tend to switch dependencies even if they stop overindulging in one activity that produces dopamine. If they do not realize that other activities will produce the same effect they will be vulnerable to repeating the same problem over and over. People who do that often mistakenly think they have an addictive personality. Experiencing a rush from extreme behavior will encourage people to live in extreme ways.

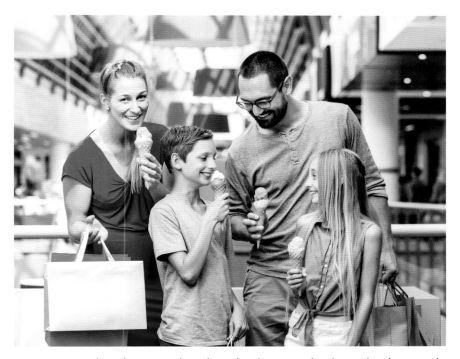

Fig. 2.12. Without knowing about how the dopamine levels can be decreased, increased, and flooded in their systems, people often bounce between various substances and activities in search of the same high—here a family enjoys ice cream while out on a shopping spree.

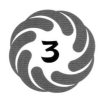

Using Your Head Too Much Can Drive You Out of Your Mind

LINEAR THINKING AND POWER STRUGGLES

Our ways of thinking about life can also contribute to our feeling overwhelmed. It is easy to forget that—while logic and rationality can play a big role in certain aspects of life like mathematics and business—interactions between a person and his or her environment are more governed by cycles. Since we each have the ability to have our own unique perspective on situations and also because we can each focus on different aspects of a situation, we can each come to our own unique opinions about the same set of circumstances. As a result, we can easily argue with each other about who has the right opinion. It is also true that two people can be on opposite sides of an issue and both be right.

For example, a couple might be arguing about whether or not one of them is going to the bar too often. For the sake of simple description, let us say that the accused person in this case is the husband. The husband then might complain that the reason he goes to the bar is because his spouse is nagging him too much. His wife could argue back that she is nagging him because he keeps going to the bar. Who is right? They are probably both right. However, they are negatively feeding off of each other. They are actually each contributing to making their situation worse. They are responding to their situation as if there is only one right answer and only one solution and so they try to overpower the other person with their logic. The situation becomes a power struggle over who is right when in fact they are both right. Instead of working together to restore the bond between them and transform their fears about what is happening to their relationship, they react to each other from a position of self-righteousness and end up in a vicious cycle that they cannot resolve. They both become more extreme in reaction to what the other person is saying and doing as they struggle with each other. Staying in that frustrating dynamic eventually feels overwhelming.

It is easy for that dynamic to get started and difficult to know how to sort it out. If you want to experience something similar in a safe way, get a tissue box and hold one end. Give the other end of the box to someone else. Explain that the box represents the bond between the two of you. Then pretend that the two of you seem to be on opposite sides of some issue. You both have valid points to support your point of view and you both would like to convince the other person to agree with your side of the argument. To physically illustrate that desire to convince each other, you will each pull on the tissue box and try to get the other person to come toward you. As soon as the other person starts pulling, you will likely pull more on your end so as not to lose your hold. That prompts the other person to pull as well, and soon you have a power struggle in which you both are pulling harder than you intended at the beginning of the exercise. Keep in mind that you are now struggling over a tissue box and there really is no particular topic that is at the heart of the power struggle. The box might even tear at some point from the strain it is under, which represents the bond between the two of you breaking.

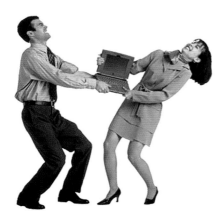

Fig. 3.1. Power struggles are easy to get into and often difficult to resolve peacefully.

Why did this happen? Is it because you are bad people? No. Is it because you have huge, unrealistic needs for control? No. It is just because you are both human beings. We all have the ability to focus on different aspects of the same issue and do not like to be told how to view them. This kind of bind can happen in lots of different ways. People can struggle over whether or not to continue an argument, whether or not they should get married, whether or not someone should be confronted about their behavior, who should have control of the money in the household, or whether or not they should have sex. We can even have internal power struggles. We all experience feeling conflicted at times. An example of an internal struggle might occur at a dance for teenagers. A youngster might be anxious to ask someone special to dance but might also feel an inner compulsion to just play it safe and ask someone who is most likely going to say yes.

How do you get out of a power struggle? In the example of pulling on a tissue box, if you pull harder, trying to force the other person or the other part of yourself that you want to control, the struggle will likely continue. If you drop your end of the box, which in real-life situations would be just giving in to the other person or the opposing urge inside of you, the risk is that the other person or an old bad habit will win and you will walk away feeling defeated or resentful. Fear, pride, and our need for control keep us locked in position. Now try easing up on your grip on the box. Usually the other person will automatically ease up as well. Then you can relax more and so can the other person, and eventually you are both just holding the box comfortably. In other words, feelings are the bottom line in human interactions, not being right.

This works with a power struggle over a tissue box and a nonexistent topic, but how do you sort it out when the topic is real and personal between you and someone whose opinion is important to you? How do you resolve the warring impulses inside yourself? This challenge will be addressed more completely when we present the technique that has been created to kick-start and encourage your natural internal processing system. For now you can start by relaxing, recognizing that control will not always be possible, looking for ways in which to concede a point, finding areas in which opposing points of view can agree, and looking for ways to compromise.

We tend not to be trained for relationship dynamics in everyday circles. Most of our learning about how to deal with life comes from our parents, school, and friends, none of which are likely to understand how relationships work unless they work in the psychology field. Without knowledge of how cycles and paradoxes play a part in our relationships with other people and with nature, we are likely to feel more and more frustrated as we struggle to conquer nature instead of working with it. For example, if you are trying to connect with someone over a sensitive issue, and the more you try to approach her or him about it, the more she or he pulls away from you, what do you do?

Black-and-White Thinking

Perhaps because we tend to need to produce the right answer at school and at work and our parents have taught us the "right" way to do things, people often develop black-and-white views of the world. This makes it seem like there is also only one way to solve problems that involve people, which of course is not true. That kind of thinking can pave the way for intolerance, judgment, and even bigotry. It also sets us up for disappointment and even for becoming overwhelmed in life because we will

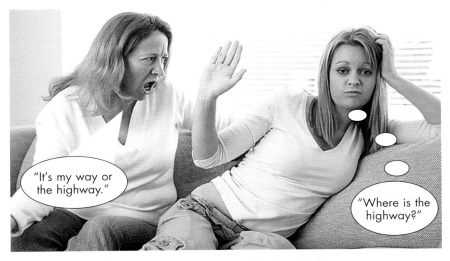

Fig. 3.2. Just because a situation seems black and white to one person does not mean it will to everyone else involved.

inevitably come across circumstances that challenge our cut-and-dried views of reality. Experiencing the exceptions to the rule in life and the gray areas of the issues that we face can be opportunities for growing, but only if people are prepared for the possibility that they exist.

In fact, life is rich with many hues and paradoxes, as Lao Tzu illustrates in chapter 2 of the Tao Te Ching:

> *In the world,*
> *Everyone recognizes beauty as beauty,*
> *Since the ugly is also there.*
> *Everyone recognizes goodness as goodness,*
> *Since evil is also there.*
> *Since being and nonbeing give birth to each other,*
> *Difficulty and ease complete each other,*
> *Long and short measure each other,*
> *High and low overflow into each other,*
> *Voice and sound harmonize with each other,*
> *And before and after follow each other.*

Therefore the sage
Lives in actionless engagement
And preaches wordless doctrine.
The myriad creatures
Act without beginning,
Nourish without possessing,
Accomplish without claiming credit.
It is accomplishment without claiming credit that
  makes the outcome Self-sustaining.

Other than reading the Tao Te Ching, or books such as *The Dance of Deception* by Harriet Goldhor Lerner, helpful guides to learning about paradoxes and cycles are rare.

NEGATIVE THINKING

Many influences teach us to search for problems and then try to sort out what solution will deal with them the most effectively: school, parents, family, friends, and mass media. Searching for problems becomes a habit and can lead to a tendency to focus on the negative. Focusing on the negative can lead to depression, anxiety, and feeling overwhelmed, robbing us of the opportunity to see and experience the positive side of situations.

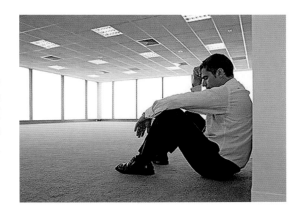

Fig. 3.3. Negative thinking can rob us of the opportunity to see and experience the positive side of the situations in our lives.

Valuing Smart, Devaluing Wisdom

Many people in modern society measure success by the acquisition of money and possessions. In many groups it is not so important how people gained those things, just as long as they have them. The wisdom that it takes to live with less and be grateful for it, to forgive people for their wrongdoings toward us, and to act in ways that protect our planet are not given as much widespread regard. Spiritual wisdom is not something that exists automatically in us. It needs to be cultivated. Those people who are not living in circumstances that encourage spiritual growth are more likely to join the "rat race" and be subject to the stresses and disappointments that are inherent in it.

As Lao Tzu says in chapter 3 of the Tao Te Ching:

> *Do not exalt intelligence and people will not*
> *compete;*
> *Do not value rare goods and people will not steal;*
> *Do not display for public view and people will not*
> *desire.*

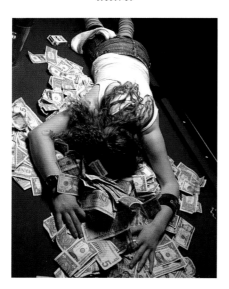 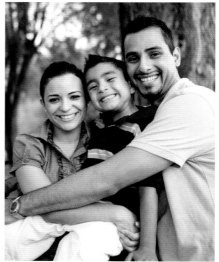

Fig. 3.4. What you believe you need and what will actually make you happy are often two very different things.

CONFUSING THE MIND
WITH THE BRAIN

Often in modern society we assume that the brain and the mind are one and the same. However, many ancient practices and even current research have acknowledged that the mind is more than just the brain. The mind represents the energy field of consciousness that we can access. The mind and the body are connected and can influence each other. The mind can also make connections with universal knowledge. Carl Jung, one of our fathers of modern psychology, called that universal knowledge the collective unconscious. When people are not aware of their mind's greater connections to universal knowledge, they downplay or ignore their intuitive knowledge and respond to life purely based on "the facts," the things that they can sense with their five sense organs. This limits their ability to live in harmony with their surroundings. They only know that they are not being effective in their lives when the evidence is obvious to them, so they are often slow to recognize when they need to change their approach.

Not Using Our Second Brain Enough

In our modern world most of us use our brains a lot. We use our brains to remember our "to do" lists and to sort out what we need to do about all the situations that life presents to us. The term "burnout" is

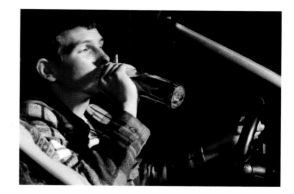

Fig. 3.5. "I don't see why people make such a big deal about drinking and driving. I've done it many times and haven't had an accident yet." Don't believe everything that you think.

commonly used in modern society. It means that the stress of dealing with our circumstances has led us to feel too tired, both physically and mentally, to carry out our normal duties. We know now that our brains can use up to 80 percent of our bodies' energy.

When we are struggling with how to best address a situation, many of our friends and family will suggest "listen to your gut instinct." In the Universal Healing Tao we emphasize the importance of working with the lower tan tien, a major energy center located about two finger-widths below the navel and three finger-widths inside the body. Current Western medical research is validating that in fact our lower abdominal area can function as a second brain. Our upper brain seems to be able to think and therefore it is better suited to remembering lists and solving mathematical equations. It has a tendency to divide our reality into pieces in order to make sense of it.

Our second brain seems to be able to think, feel, and intuit; it therefore seems better suited to sorting out how to respond to the challenges of life. The second brain can accept reality without having to subdivide it. Focusing on the second brain brings energy to the major energy center, making us less likely to experience burnout. It also brings our focus and energy to the center of the body, which helps us to feel grounded and centered. On the other hand, ignoring our gut can lead to confusion and less-than-satisfying results. (More information about the second brain and how to work with its energy can be found in *Tan Tien Chi Kung* by Mantak Chia.)

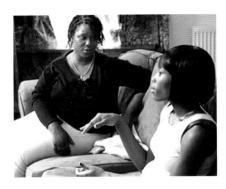

Fig. 3.6. "I caught him cheating again. My gut instinct tells me that I should dump him, but my head says I'll never find a guy who is perfect, especially at this stage of my life." Ignoring your gut can lead to confusion and less-than-satisfying results.

UNCONSCIOUS PROCESSES CAN DISTRACT US FROM REALITY

That's How We Roll

Our emotional states are somewhat governed by momentum. Once we have started moving, we tend to keep rolling in the same direction. For example, most of us have noticed that when we start thinking negatively, we usually continue to find more things to think negatively about after that. That type of thinking eventually creates a negative mood. If we cannot stop that tendency, negativity becomes a way of viewing the world and can lead to anger, depression, and resentment. Repetition reinforces the connection between ideas, states, and experiences. Think of it like threads that are being connected one at a time between a mood and a repeated negative thought or unhealthy activity. The threads that are thicker are the connections that have been made more often.

Denial

Many of us were raised to believe that having negative feelings is wrong or a sign of weakness. Therefore we shove our feelings down and try to ignore them in hopes that they will go away. But they do not. They pile

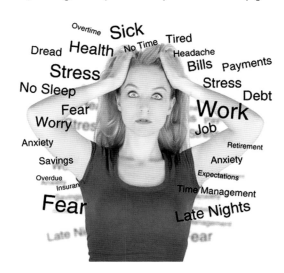

Fig. 3.7. Repeating unhealthy thoughts and habits reinforces them inside of us. Over time they can become automatic reactions that we can no longer control.

up inside of us, creating fear, worry, and resentment. Without realizing or remembering that everything and everyone is not perfect, we tend to feel ashamed of our negative feelings and try to hide them. We pretend that we are fine in public and wonder in silence why we are not "normal" like everybody else seems to be.

Denial is actually a natural process that helps us to control the amount of information about our environment that we receive at one time. If we are feeling uncomfortable it is natural to turn our focus outside of ourselves. Our denial system acts like a fuse box. The more we receive information that we do not want to acknowledge, the more the lights go out. We would hope that when we are obviously in trouble we would wake up to the reality, but often just the opposite happens. Loved ones often want to shake or scream at someone who is spiraling downward in this way, but that will just overwhelm the person even more and keep the spiral going.

In today's society there is also something developing that could be called "New Age denial." It involves acknowledging only the positive aspects of life or pretending that everything is great for fear that acknowledging anything negative will attract negative energy and negative results. That approach can create ironic results. As people try to see everything in a positive light, they are not prepared for or responding effectively to the inevitable negative things that will happen. Denial

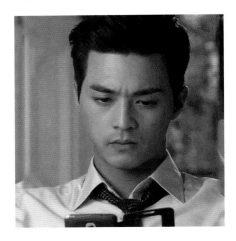

Fig. 3.8. "My wife said she's leaving me if I don't start spending more time at home. I'm sure she's just tired. My first wife was demanding like that when she was tired." When we are not prepared to see the truth of our situations we are likely in for a rude awakening later.

that goes beyond its natural purpose to protect us from overwhelming effects of life events will eventually bring on the kinds of negative results that we are trying to escape in the first place.

POOR USE OF VISUALIZATION

Many people do not realize that much of what we think about needs to be translated into pictures before we can understand it on a deeper level. Another related piece of information that many people do not have is that our bodies respond to what we visualize as if it is real regardless of whether or not the pictures in our minds fit with reality. Do you want proof of that? Picture a beautiful lake on a warm, sunny day. The sun is shining off the water. You can hear the sounds and smell the scents of nature around you. You can feel the air and the sun on your body. How do you feel? Notice that you did not have to go anywhere to feel the relaxation and contentment of that scene.

When people do not realize how visualization works, they often use it in ways that actually make their problems worse instead of better. For example, many people tell themselves to "stop" or avoid doing something, like drinking alcohol, doing illicit drugs, gambling, or doing anything else to excess. Thinking in that way forces the deeper parts of their minds to make a picture of the activity that they want to stop or avoid. Then they get rid of the picture to complete the "stop" or "don't" command. This is a confusing way to get the message across and it ends up triggering the very thing that is not wanted before the full intention of the message is communicated. Consistent repetition of that mistake can contribute to or even create obsessive thinking.

Talent for Visualization Creates Challenges

Dyslexia is a much more widespread problem than most people realize. Most people know that dyslexics often have problems with learning to read in childhood. Many people think there is only one kind of dyslexia, the kind in which a person turns letters backward when he or she

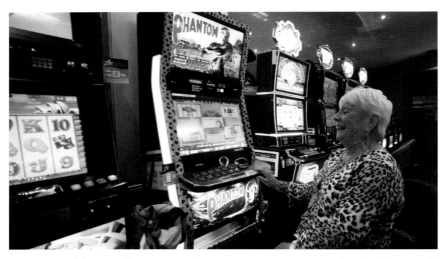

Fig. 3.9. Addictive substances and activities sometimes provide relief for people who have trouble concentrating, but of course those substances and activities can create worse problems later on.

writes. However, there are many kinds of dyslexia. Ronald Davis, the author of *The Gift of Dyslexia,* points out that people who have dyslexia have a strong ability to visualize. Since some of our words, such as *a, an,* and *the,* do not have visual translations, they create stumbling blocks for people who have dyslexia. This type of challenge can create frustration all through life for people who do not realize why they are struggling or how to work around it. If those frustrations and disappointments are not resolved, they can pile up inside people to the point where the emotional weight of them becomes overwhelming.

Some addictive substances and activities, like cocaine and gambling, seem to provide a sense of greater focus for people who have dyslexia. That feeling of greater focus can strongly reinforce the idea of continuing to use those things.

MISUNDERSTANDING TRANCE

Depictions of trance in movies, television shows, and hypnosis stage shows has unfortunately given the public some faulty impressions about trance and its uses. People generally have the impression that trance is something that is difficult to achieve and only experts in the field can accomplish it. However, anyone can achieve a trance state. It is also commonly believed that hypnotists have unlimited power over their subjects. Actually all hypnosis is self-hypnosis, so a hypnotist is just someone who leads the subject through the process of accessing a trance state. Trance is achieved when there is a blending of conscious and unconscious levels of awareness, not just accessing unconscious ones. Since the conscious mind is still accessible, people will not do things that they are opposed to doing, even when they are in a trance state.

Some people believe they cannot go into a trance state because they are too intelligent or strong-willed, but the truth is we all go into trance every day. A common example of this is when we are about to go to sleep. At that time we often know we are close to going to sleep. Our bodies are relaxed and warm and do not feel like moving much, and our minds are wandering from conscious thought to something like a daydream stream of consciousness. That is trance. The conscious and unconscious minds are intermingling. Another common example is when we walk or drive somewhere and then realize that we cannot

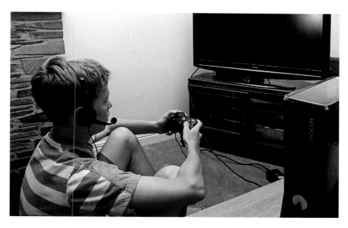

Fig 3.10. Not understanding how vulnerable we are when our mental guard is down can make us vulnerable to some addictive activities.

remember all the things that we did to get there because our minds were wandering during the trip.

It is actually easy to go into trance. Our conscious minds are only built to hold about seven to nine pieces of information at a time. If we try to hold on to more than that, our dreaming minds tend to come forward and we go into trance. Think about a child in school who is becoming overwhelmed with the amount of information that is being offered in a class. He or she eventually starts daydreaming or looking out the window. Imagine now how easily people can go into trance with the amount of information that our modern lifestyles provide. Once we are in a trance state we are more suggestible, so our ability to think critically about the messages we receive from other people and mass media is reduced. If we do not know how to use trance to train the deeper parts of our minds to fight against unwanted influences or propel us toward our goals, we are more likely to have difficulty taking charge of our lives in healthy and productive ways.

HEALTH VS. NARCISSISM

Lao Tzu reminds us in chapter 22 of the Tao Te Ching:

> *Those who boast of themselves lose their stance.*
> *He who displays himself is not seen.*
> *He who justifies himself is not understood.*
> *He who lashes out does not succeed.*
> *He who builds himself up does not endure.*
> *In the sense of Tao,*
> *This is said to be eating too much and acting too much.*
> *It results in disgust.*
> *Those who desire will not endure.*

However, in order to not be accused of being egotistical or "having a swelled head," many of us have developed a habit of not openly

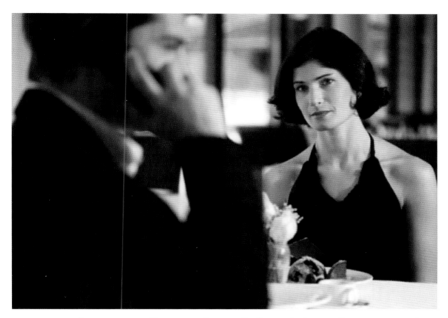

Fig. 3.11. If we cannot allow ourselves to feel good about who we are in the moment, we tend to add external sources of distraction and enjoyment.

acknowledging our best qualities or accomplishments. That can become a habit to the point where we automatically downplay or ignore our shining moments and subtly or openly reject praise or compliments from the people around us. This can limit our self-esteem and increase the likelihood that we will have to turn to some other, external source to help us feel good. Many external things that

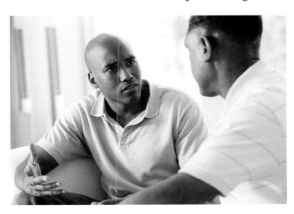

Fig. 3.12. "How did you get a raise?" The other one says, "I just explained to him that I'm the best worker in the office over and over until he believed me."

we buy and do will eventually become boring and not enjoyable over time. This can lead to us continually searching for the next best thing to make us feel good instead of just enjoying being alive and celebrating our successes.

In our competitive and materialistic world the people who are good at self-promotion have an edge. People who are humble are not as good at it. Narcissism is rewarded and celebrated as a result. Narcissism involves having an overdeveloped sense of self that masks underlying insecurity. Material advantages for narcissists can distract them from the emotional pain that would otherwise push them to rebalance their egos. Humility stands between low self-esteem and narcissism.

THE PROBLEM WITH PERFECTIONISM

Many people do not realize that their approach to life is perfectionistic. They think that being a perfectionist means that a person does everything perfectly. That is not a perfectionist. That is a perfect person. Perfectionism means that a person does not allow himself or herself to feel satisfied or take credit for his or her accomplishments until they have been completed or done perfectly.

Many people are raised to believe that the best way to motivate themselves to achieve their goals is to do their best and not be satis-

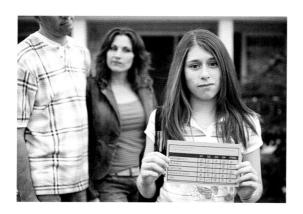

Fig. 3.13. Her father says, "Oh well, maybe you'll do better next year." She thinks to herself, "I'll never be good enough."

fied until they have accomplished perfection in their chosen area. That sounds good on the surface, but it does not allow for celebration along the way to achieving the goal or giving oneself credit if the best that can be achieved is partial accomplishment of the goal. Perfectionism can be a set-up. People who adopt such an approach are inevitably going to find that they cannot always do things perfectly. Then they are vulnerable to developing low self-esteem or even self-loathing, which increases the likelihood that they will eventually get depressed.

Perfectionism can also lead to feeling flawed or unworthy deep inside, even when others see you as someone who "has it all together." It creates an increase of anxiety that may not even be recognized. That can lead to becoming critical of others and yourself because you are searching for a reason why you do not feel right no matter how hard you try. Looking outward can prevent you from realizing your deep-seated feelings of shame. Shame makes it difficult for you to be accountable, to learn lessons from your experiences.

When shame is combined with perfectionism, you can feel an internal power struggle between wanting to be perfect and wanting to change nothing at all. The tension between those two extremes can halt your progress. You become afraid to fail and afraid to be anything other than perfect. Meanwhile you cannot help but notice your lack of progress or mastery. This often reinforces negative beliefs that you have formed about yourself.

The sage, as described by Lao Tzu in chapter 73 of the Tao Te Ching, offers us a wiser example:

> *Knowing that you don't know [everything] is*
> *superior.*
> *Not knowing that you don't know [everything]*
> *is a sickness.*
> *So the sage's being without sickness is that he*
> *knows sickness as sickness;*
> *Thus, he is without sickness.*

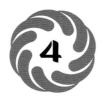

Trauma and Addiction Keep People from "Living the Good Life"

THE TRAUMA OF EXPERIENCES THAT ARE TOO HARD TO SWALLOW

Are there things that have happened in your past that still bother you now and you wish they didn't? Some energy is just too dark and heavy to easily dissolve. Sometimes we have experiences in life that are too awful, too strange, or too terrible to process away easily. Some of what happens in life is "too hard to swallow," as the old saying goes. Since many of us do not know how to process our emotions effectively and thoroughly in the first place, it is also possible for our emotions to pile up over time, creating a dark, heavy, toxic emotional weight that is too big to process, even though the events making up the pile were not that extreme to begin with. Either way, at a certain point too much dark and heavy energy becomes stuck inside, overloading the ability of our natural emotional processing systems to cope.

When people become overwhelmed they often become polarized inside. They automatically separate the incident from their view of themselves. They make a division between "me" and "not me." How-

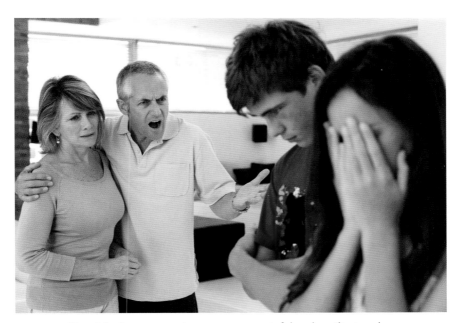

Fig. 4.1. Some experiences are so painful or humiliating that
we are not able to accept them.

ever, deep down inside they often wonder or believe that if they were
somehow a better person then the problem would not have occurred.
This seemingly leaves people with the option of either continuing to
make that separation and feeling like victims with some underlying guilt
or shame, or acknowledging that the problem arose because they were
somehow lacking as a person. Neither option is particularly appealing,
so they often end up vacillating between the two without resolution,
sometimes believing that the issue is a reflection of them as human
beings, and sometimes feeling like victims. The issue becomes stuck
inside them because there seems to be no viable way to sort it out. This
whole process happens beyond the conscious awareness of the affected
person. The undigested experience takes up energetic space inside the
person.

For example, children who are sexually abused often judge themselves as being bad or dirty. If the suffering they have undergone as a
result of the abuse is compassionately validated by others who matter to

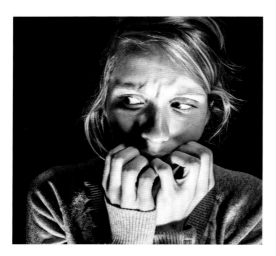

Fig. 4.2. Toxic feelings connected to overwhelming events from our past can become a dark, heavy energy in and around us.

them, that helps them to process it and experience themselves as "normal." On the other hand, if important friends or relatives tell them it did not happen, or it did not happen in that way, or blame them, it is more likely that they will end up feeling worse.

WHAT WATER TELLS US

Masaru Emoto, a Japanese researcher, is famous for his books about messages from water. He has systematically exposed water molecules to different spoken phrases that are either positive or negative, and then photographed what happens to the water molecules. The changes in the water molecules are dramatic. His research suggests that what we think

Fig. 4.3. Human beings are mostly water. Our water molecules are dramatically affected by how we think about and talk to ourselves.

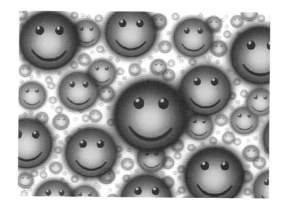

about ourselves and life in general has a profound effect on how we are functioning on a molecular level.

Polarities and Comparisons

In order to understand how we process experiences and how toxic or overwhelming ones become stuck inside us, a new concept needs to be introduced at this point. The concept is called "polarities." In Taoism they are expressed as yin and yang, which refer to the duality of our experience of reality. We experience life as composed of various pairs of opposites like black and white, positive and negative, hard and soft. Taoism teaches that both aspects of life are inherent to our existence. We need the black side to appreciate and understand the white side. However, few people have the helpful perspective of the Tao Te Ching, chapter 28:

> *Understanding the male and holding on to the*
> *female*
> *Enables the flow of the world.*
> *This being the flow of the world, the eternal action*
> *abides.*
> *Knowing that the eternal action abides is to return*
> *to childhood.*
> *Understanding the pure and holding on to the*
> *impure*
> *Enables the cleansing of the world.*
> *With the cleansing of the world, ongoing action*
> *suffices.*
> *When ongoing action suffices, it returns to*
> *simplicity.*
> *Understanding the white and holding on to the*
> *black*
> *Enables the formation of the world.*
> *Being the formation of the world, ongoing action*
> *does not stray.*

When ongoing action does not stray, it returns to
  the infinite.
This simplicity takes shape as a mechanism.
The sage makes it the head ruler.
Great ruling never divides.

We make comparisons in order to understand the world around us. As we make comparisons between our past and present, present and future, ideal world and reality, ideal self and actual self, and every other experience we have, we have the potential to find similarities and differences. As we unconsciously swing like a pendulum between the two elements, we can figure out how they are similar and different, until they seem like a new concept that can be compared to some other new experience.

Incidentally, this concept could be extended to help understand why even though there are over two hundred formally recognized approaches to psychotherapy, many research studies have found that they are basically equally effective. The polarities concept may suggest that each of those approaches, consciously or not, is addressing a different polarity. For example, psychoanalysis could be addressing the past versus present polarity, while cognitive-behavioral therapy may be focusing more on the thoughts versus feelings polarity.

Polarities form between our existing knowledge and new experiences. Our natural tendency is to try to explore the new experience until it connects with our existing knowledge. For example, when we meet someone new we often notice our differences from that person at first. Over time, however, as we get to know that person we discover more and more similarities until "you" and "I" seem more like "we." And then "we" can be compared to other people that we meet next.

Symptoms of Too Much Emotional Baggage

When people feel overwhelmed by something that has happened to them or around them it changes their perspective on life. It also seems to open them up to other levels of awareness, but they often do not know how to control that awareness. They are more aware of how fragile life is and sometimes they can connect with others on a level that is deeper than most people can achieve. Such awareness can be a real gift once they learn how to accept it and work with it. Until then, though, it just makes them even more affected by what goes on around them.

When people carry heavy emotional burdens they feel the weight of them. They often feel fragile, weak, and overly sensitive, cycling between depression and anxiety as they struggle to keep functioning in their daily lives. Just as with a heavy physical weight, people will eventually collapse under the weight of heavy emotional energy. Even if they later pick themselves up again, they may continue feeling anxious because they know that they could collapse again. The heaviness of the past is still weighing them down. It is not their fault. They are not flawed or "damaged goods." They are simply feeling the natural effects of being overwhelmed by life and the emotional toll of their experiences has become so significant that it has now become physical. The immaterial has become material.

If the energy becomes dense and heavy enough, their ability to

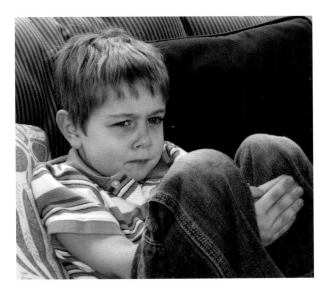

Fig. 4.4. Unresolved feelings clog up and stall our emotional processing system.

transform or expel the toxins will not be able to function anymore. They become like an engine with a clogged carburetor or a stream that is dammed up. Eventually what goes on inside them becomes too uncomfortable. Without knowing any other way to deal with the discomfort, they start to take their attention off of their bodies and focus more on their thoughts. They start to lose touch with what is going on inside them and begin to rely more and more on suppressing and denying their emotional and physical pain to manage their internal world.

THE INTERPLAY BETWEEN TRAUMA AND ADDICTION

Spiraling Further Downward

Each time a person who has had a traumatic experience has new ones that are similar, the negative energy seems to pile onto the initial experience emotionally and energetically, creating even darker and heavier baggage in the person. If that happens often enough, the person will feel weighed down emotionally, physically, and spiritually. This can create clinical depression and anxiety disorders.

If a person does not know or learn how to balance that energy and instead comes across an addictive substance or activity that seems to temporarily relieve symptoms and distract from the memory of traumatic incidents, then she or he is vulnerable to developing an addiction as well. Some people go toward stimulants like gambling, nicotine, coffee, or cocaine, while others tend to go toward "downers" like alcohol, pain-killing prescription drugs, or heroin. The effect of having the symptoms suddenly removed makes a big impression on people. It is a very compelling effect. However, it is like the Trojan horse: the solution looks great at first, but after the effect wears off, it brings more problems with it than were there in the first place. The dark energy taxes the entire energetic system and people become progressively more tired. Then they are more likely to gravitate toward more quick fixes.

The more people become involved with something addictive, the

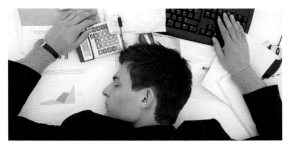

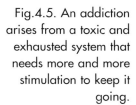

Fig.4.5. An addiction arises from a toxic and exhausted system that needs more and more stimulation to keep it going.

more likely it is they will turn to other addictive activities to address their mood as they tire and crash. Think about the extreme example of people living on the streets. Often they are seen drinking coffee, smoking, and eating fast food. People are essentially good when their internal systems are healthy and clean, but they exhibit more and more addictive behavior as their energetic systems become toxic.

Addiction Drains the Body

We are born with a certain limited amount of energy. Half of our energy is set aside as our daily energy. Our kidneys carry 25 percent of our energy for life. The other 25 percent is stored in the sexual organs. As a person becomes weighted down by unprocessed emotions and experiences, and then uses something addictive to manage that weight, his or her internal organs become unbalanced and weaker. The body responds to the presence of the addictive substance or the effects of an addictive activity as a poison, so it sends out something akin to a yellow alert signal, which activates the adrenal glands. It tricks the body into creating a fight-or-flight response. The adrenal glands then send a message to the kidneys to produce more energy. That feels great at the time but after it wears off the person feels exhausted.

If the person does not know how to regain energy in a healthy way, or the pattern has become too engrained, she or he will return to the addictive substance or activity. That cycle drains the person more and more. The sexual energy drains out first. Then once the sexual organs are drained of their chi, energy is drawn from the kidneys. If the kidneys are drained, energy will start to drain from the brain. Then the person will have difficulty thinking clearly, which increases the likelihood that she or he will make unhealthy choices. This is why so many famous people in the entertainment industry die young. We cheer them on and celebrate when they use up tremendous amounts of energy to entertain us. However, they cannot keep up that energy level forever. They inevitably need to turn to artificial stimulation to maintain that level of energetic output. From there they are subject to the same perils that would happen to anyone else. As Lao Tzu puts it in chapter 44 of the Tao Te Ching:

> *Which is more cherished, the name or the body?*
> *Which is worth more, the body or possessions?*
> *Which is more beneficial, to gain or to lose?*
> *Extreme fondness is necessarily very costly.*
> *The more you cling to, the more you lose.*
> *So knowing what is sufficient averts disgrace.*
> *Knowing when to stop averts danger.*
> *This can lead to a longer life.*

Once the kidneys become drained, the other organs are drawn into the process in the destructive cycle until they are all out of balance and full of toxins. At that point the negative emotions and states that are produced by each organ are all present: hastiness, impatience, hatred, and cruelty from the heart; negative thinking, overthinking, and worry from the spleen; grief, sadness, loss, and depression from the lungs; fear,

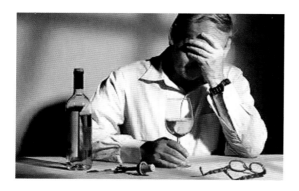

Fig. 4.6. Addiction drains the kidneys, sexual organs, and the brain.

anxiety, phobias, and trauma from the kidneys; and anger, frustration, jealousy, envy, and shame from the liver. This is the personality cluster that the 12-step community refers to as "Slick": a reminder for people that who they are when their systems are clean, sober, and balanced is not the same as when they are active in their addictions.

When a person is triggered by a person, place, or situation that reminds him or her of the memory that is connected to the unresolved energy inside, it brings up emotions again, which triggers the whole yellow alert process all over again. That process can produce a rapid decline in that person and make it very difficult to find the energy to make healthy changes using willpower alone.

The weight of the unresolved energy also tends to create an automatic response in which the personality is split in order to protect the person from unwanted feelings and memories. Then the overwhelming experiences are contained in only a portion of her or his identity and the rest of the psyche remains intact. However, the splits obstruct the

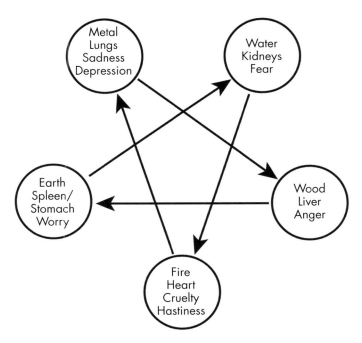

Fig. 4.7. Destructive cycle of the internal organs

communication between the different aspects of the personality. This leads the person to communicate in confusing and compulsive ways and experience consequences that do not make sense to him or her.

Repetitive actions, obsessive thoughts, and compulsions that are continually fed will eventually plough energetic pathways in the body, which become denser and stronger until the body accepts them as a new part of the body. This encodes a new energetic tattoo of sorts inside the person's energetic matrix. That tattoo has a new agenda based on the toxic energy of each of the imbalanced and toxic organs. In contrast and often in opposition to the intentions of the person it inhabits, the addictive hologram lies, cheats, manipulates, and steals, and acts in self-destructive ways. Those acts are often referred to as addictive behavior in the recovery community. The emotional processing system that is handled by the internal organs is out of balance and full of toxins. The person cannot emotionally grow until that system has been restored to health.

Crash

Getting to the point where a person cannot stand living in such an unhealthy way anymore is what is commonly referred to as "hitting rock bottom" in the recovery community. While a person is still medicating his or her feelings with the addictive substance or activity, the urgency to make healthy changes is prevented from building to the point where it forces the person to take action. In the meantime the person cannot emotionally mature, so even when he or she is not actively involved with something addictive, his or her behavior seems inappropriate, chaotic,

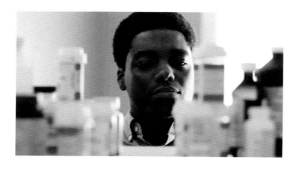

Fig. 4.8. As addiction progresses it gets worse. People eventually create a lifestyle in which uppers and downers are routinely used to manage their moods.

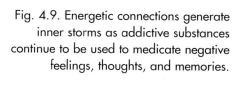

Fig. 4.9. Energetic connections generate inner storms as addictive substances continue to be used to medicate negative feelings, thoughts, and memories.

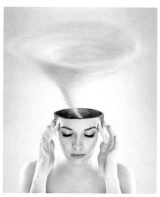

and disorganized. The person's system tries to clean out the toxins and rebalance itself, which takes extra effort. That extra effort creates friction and heat. Heat rises and gets stuck in the brain. As a result people who are afflicted in this way have trouble concentrating and calming down.

Without knowledge of how to manage their emotions in healthy ways, people tend to alternate between using stimulating and numbing addictive substances and activities. They develop a pattern or ritual of using uppers and downers of various kinds in an attempt to create a cocktail of balance. However, that cocktail creates the opposite effect. It only increases the size of the swing toward extreme emotions. We can see this pattern starting to develop in a person who uses cigarettes or coffee during the day for energy and alcohol or prescription drugs at night to calm down and get to sleep.

The unresolved energy can affect people on all levels. Often on a less than completely conscious level, they develop negative and irrational beliefs about themselves, such as "I'm a screw-up," "I don't deserve to be happy," "I'm no good," "I can't stand up for myself," and "It was my fault." It affects them emotionally, too, so that they feel upset when they think about the incidents connected to the energy and they feel less connected to everyday life the rest of the time. It can affect them physically in the sense that they feel pain or tension in certain points or areas of the body whenever the issue comes to mind.

Each time a person experiences something similar to the memories that are stored in those addiction pathways, she or he may have urges, thoughts, or cravings to return to the addiction. In the recovery community those events are called "triggers." When the person is no longer able to consistently resist those urges, he or she is considered addicted and will require an extensive overhaul of his or her lifestyle to effectively work around that set of pathways. Addiction is a continuum, too. People who feed their addiction more heavily over a longer period of time have even more work to do to reverse that process enough to regain control over their lives.

Meanwhile, it is difficult for the people around them to understand how these individuals have become so unhealthy and ineffective in life, so they tend to judge them. They are often referred to as "losers" and "quitters." Even in active addiction, people still feel the judgment and condemnation of those around them. It does not wake them up to the reality of their predicament, as some people would hope. On the contrary, it reinforces the guilt and shame that they already feel and even adds to it, which creates even more emotional baggage for them to clear out before they can become the kind of person who would not be judged like that.

The pileup of blockages in their systems limits their feelings of well-being and faith in themselves. Without knowing how to reconnect to whatever kind of faith they used to have, or even knowing that they

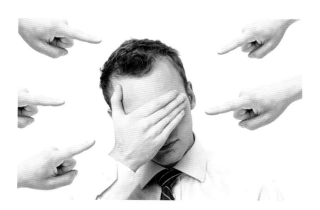

Fig. 4.10. People who are struggling with an addiction are often judged. The experience of being judged only adds to the shame that they are trying to medicate through using something addictive.

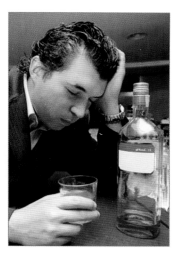

Fig. 4.11. As people become more and more dependent on something addictive, their faith that anything else can help them becomes progressively weaker.

need to reconnect, they become increasingly focused on external solutions. That external focus leads to more pile-up.

DYNAMICS OF ADDICTION

Codependency

People who are concerned about someone who has an addiction tend to develop certain tendencies, especially if the addicted people are directly affecting their lives with the consequences of their behavior. "Codependency" refers to the tendency of people to put the needs of others before themselves and to try to control people through manipulation. They also tend to worry about the addicted people and that becomes a habit.

It is like they are riding in the same car as the addicted person and the addict is driving all over the road. The natural tendency is to try to grab hold of the wheel or to yell at the driver to be more careful. Such people end up obsessing over a person in much the same way as an addicted person obsesses over a drug or an activity. There is a saying in the recovery community that "Underneath every addict is a codependent." When their moods are chemically altered and they are in denial, people with addictions tend to think that other people are the source of

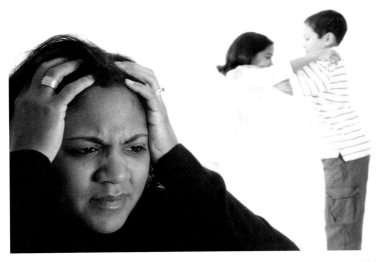

Fig. 4.12. Focusing on others too much and neglecting oneself leads to resentment. Resentment can eat away at you until your system demands relief.

their problems and try to get them to change. Of course we cannot force people to change if they do not want to, so that approach is doomed and will ultimately lead to further worry, frustration, and resentment.

People who have addictions also develop a tendency to try to control things that are not within their grasp. That tendency often stems from expectations about how life "should" operate in their minds. When life does not comply, and it usually does not, people can get frustrated and resentful. Resentments can eat away at a person's emotional state and spirit for years if they are not addressed. Of course, if that happens, it is only a matter of time until a person will want to feed or return to his or her addiction to get some relief.

"Opposite Nancy"

With their energetic pathways so clogged up, dark, and slow, and their organs so weakened, people end up acting opposite to the ways that they normally would, even when they are not actively feeding their addictions. They also become more reactive when other people try to get them to change. The term "opposite Nancy" refers to the tendency of people who have addictions to do the opposite of what people tell them to do, especially people who are in positions of authority over them. Sometimes the traumas that played a part in the development of addictions in people involved an authority figure. Sometimes people have long histories in which people have tried to mold them into something that they were not and they resent that. That kind of reactivity can even be fostered when they resent people who are trying to get them to seek help when they are not ready.

Chronically Unique

Even though people who are addicted can experience denial, they are aware on some level that they seem to be functioning differently than a lot of the people around them. However, they often seem unaware that their unique aspects are similar to those of everyone else who has an addiction. They are also often unaware that many of the effects of their addictive behavior can be reversed. After people stop feeding their addictions their cells may take up to two years to repair themselves. Proper cleansing and rebalancing of their systems can help them to bring the virtues back from their organs. Without awareness of those realities they tend to expect special or unique treatment from others to help them deal with their "unique" needs. That tends to bring out frustration and resentment in others and can lead to arguments and power struggles, which might lead recovering addicts to return to unhealthy or addictive methods to make themselves feel better.

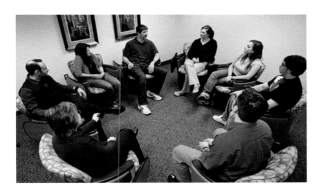

Fig. 4.13. "Chronically unique" refers to the tendency of people who have addictions to believe that their situation is too different to be helped by the same treatments and solutions that help other people.

Not Understanding "Petting the Dragon"

"Petting the dragon" is another phrase from the 12-step community. It refers to the risk of sparking urges to return to addictive activities by doing things that seem unrelated. For example, when people have gambling problems with a specific game like slot machines, they often assume that they can safely play other gambling games like the lottery or poker because they do not have a problem with them. It is not that playing those games will become a new problem. However, slot machines and the other games are conceptually connected, a connection that can be invigorated on an unconscious level by playing those other games. Then they have the desire to return to the slot machines.

Without understanding how this works people can find recovery from an addiction to be a really confusing struggle. They often blame themselves for continuing to slip back to their addictive behaviors and

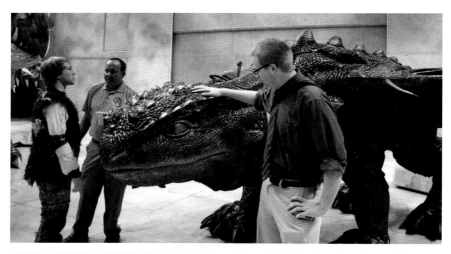

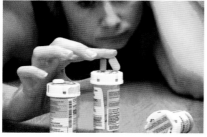

Fig. 4.14. "Petting the dragon" warns that substituting one addiction with a seemingly less dangerous one can wake up the desire to return to the original addiction.

judge themselves as weak or stupid. They feel ashamed, which gives them another negative feeling that is piling up inside them. Ironically, that pileup contributes to the desire to go back to the addictive activity, to do something that will make them feel better.

Not Understanding the Post-Acute Withdrawal Syndrome

Detoxification from an addiction can involve physical pain, nausea, sweating, headaches, vomiting, sleep disturbance, tiredness, and irritability. Many people think of the detoxification process from an addiction as something that happens within a few days to a few weeks after the active addiction is stopped. However, there are aftershock effects that continue to crop up for approximately two years. The aftershocks and the times that they occur are called the "post-acute withdrawal syndrome." They tend to occur at combinations of three and six after people stop feeding their addictions. Three weeks, six weeks, three months, six months, a year, and two years tend to be typical times when people experience these effects.

At those times people do not always have direct urges to return to their addiction. Instead they often just feel "off," irritable, and unhappy. Once people are aware of the concept it is easy to see it in action. You may have known people who have quit smoking, for example, and then one day said something like, "I don't know what happened. I was doing great for about three weeks there and then I started again." The 12-step program uses the acronym RID to stand for "restless, irritable, and discontent." The feelings from the post-acute withdrawal syndrome are temporary and will pass in a few days if people can recognize what they are and ride them out. If they do not understand what is happening, they may be led back to their addiction to make those bad feelings go away.

Trading One Rush for Another

People sometimes notice that their current lifestyle is creating too many problems for them and decide to make a change. However,

Maybe it's time you switched!

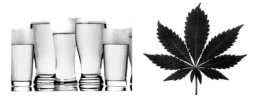

Fig. 4.15. It is easy to stop one addiction and start another.

without fully understanding how they have become conditioned toward addictive behavior, they just switch one addictive activity for another. Some people develop a problem with alcohol and then throw themselves into their work to get away from alcohol, only to find later that they have become workaholics. Another example would be when someone stops smoking cigarettes and then starts routinely overeating. This kind of unhealthy substitution perpetuates the pileup of toxins in the body. People do not realize that what they need to do is give those toxins a chance to leave their systems and then recondition their bodies to get used to natural highs, like the kind that comes from having a good laugh, instead of trying to replace one kind of extreme high with another.

Potentially Addictive Things Are Everywhere

For those people who are searching for an external source that can even temporarily give them internal peace, there are unfortunately a variety of readily available options. Even if we only limit our focus to alcohol, illicit drugs, various kinds of gambling, caffeine, and cigarettes, it becomes obvious that there are many ways to develop an addiction in our societies. Greater availability increases the likelihood that people will experiment with and eventually become dependent on something that will ultimately rob them of their inner peace.

Energetic Genetics

There has been some research evidence to support the notion that there can be a genetic predisposition for addictions, especially for alcohol addiction. However, the genetic aspect might be even more complicated and pervasive than that research indicates. Bruce Lipton, the author of the book *The Biology of Belief,* shows through his systematic research that not only can our genes affect the way we think but the beliefs that people have can also affect our genes. By applying that notion to addictions we could theorize that the beliefs that an addicted parent has could affect the beliefs that his or her child develops before the child is even born. If that is true then the effects of our modern lifestyle on parents can increase the chances that their descendants will become addicted.

DEALING WITH THE CYCLES OF TRAUMA AND ADDICTION

After reading about all of the cycles that can contribute to an addiction you might feel your head spinning and wonder how any of us can escape what the 12-step community calls the "slippery slope" into addiction. However, if we look at it another way, knowing that we are all at least a little bit on the path to—or back to—an addiction, that can help us not to be lulled into a false sense of invincibility or superiority. We all go through things that are hard for us to get over. No one is perfectly healthy. We can't simply say that either a person is addicted or not addicted, depressed or not depressed. It is a matter of to what degree each of us is on the way to developing those problems or falling back into them.

In everyday conversations people do not usually understand all of the factors and dynamics that are involved in these issues. They also have their own busy lives to attend to and do not want to get weighed down with other people's problems. As a result, people will often say something like "Awww, let it go" or "Why don't you just stop?" Well, that sounds easy, doesn't it? It is amazing how often we talk like that without having a clear way to make it as simple in practice as it sounds in theory.

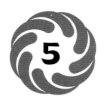

A Fragmented View of Nature Leads to Ineffective Problem Solving

Many solutions are offered to the pileup of toxins in our systems, but many of them reflect the same "divide and conquer" mentality that created the pileup in the first place.

LACK OF KNOWLEDGE OF THE TRUE NATURE OF REALITY

You might ask yourself why there does not seem to be widespread recognition of the problems that have been listed so far and why we do not have more effective treatments for them. It seems important to recognize that most of our society still operates according to Newtonian physics. Many people forget that quantum physics has been recognized since the time of Albert Einstein. Many systems of thought and healing, including the Universal Healing Tao, have operated in ways that are consistent with quantum physics for thousands of years. Despite

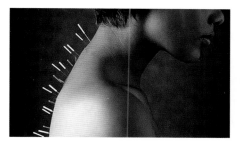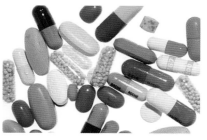

Fig. 5.1. Many so-called alternative healing systems have been around for millennia, but our societal focus on modern medicine sometimes leads people to miss out on what the other approaches have to offer.

that, modern society generally still treats the world around us as if it is solid matter, even though we have known for almost a century that all matter is energy, that matter can act as a particle or a wave depending on the expectations of the person who is experiencing it, and that time and space are just concepts that we understand due to how our senses interpret reality.

Without widespread awareness and recognition of the true nature of reality, we keep treating our health as purely a reflection of the concrete aspects of our bodies and our sanity as a reflection of the functioning of our brains. As a result, our solutions tend to involve drugs and surgery. We use concrete solutions to address a concrete version of reality. Maintaining that concrete view of reality leaves control of our health in the hands of the recognized experts and reduces our ability to empower ourselves to use preventive measures in our daily lives.

Lack of Awareness of Science, Spirituality, and their Connections

Science and spirituality now agree that all things are connected, that there is an organizing force that affects them all, and that our minds affect the energy around and within us. This knowledge can help us to understand the value of practices such as Chi Kung, but if we lack that knowledge, we might not know why we should have a spiritual practice.

If you are interested in learning more about that connection, check out the DVD called *What the Bleep Do We Know?!*

Many people view spirituality and religion as being one and the same. They may reject both if they have had unpleasant experiences with religion. However, they do not have to be the same. Spirituality can involve learning about the energetic connections between all living things and how to work with those energies, without claiming knowledge of who or what created or controls those energies. Some people view themselves as being more like scientists and reject spirituality without realizing that science and spirituality can point to similar realities. Without such an understanding, they can be deprived of their capacity

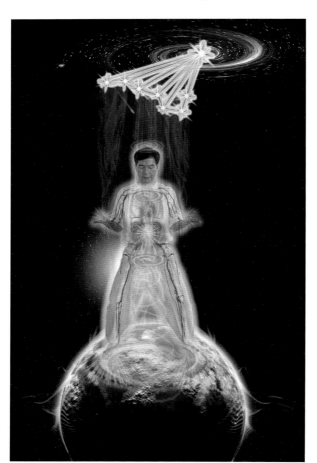

Fig. 5.2. Spirituality can involve learning about the energetic connections between all living things and how to work with those energies.

to view events in their lives as helpful or meaningful; they do not have a way to view their futures with hope and positivity. That can lead to a feeling of being disconnected from other people and a victim of random and senseless painful events in life. Then it is just a matter of time until they become overwhelmed by the pileup of painful experiences that they cannot meaningfully accept or understand. Eventually they will need to find ways to relieve those feelings, which usually leads to something addictive.

Separating Mind, Body, and Spirit

In an effort to isolate the areas that we need to heal or manage and to make the healing process simpler and more precise, professionals and laypeople have separated the mind, body, and spirit and tried to

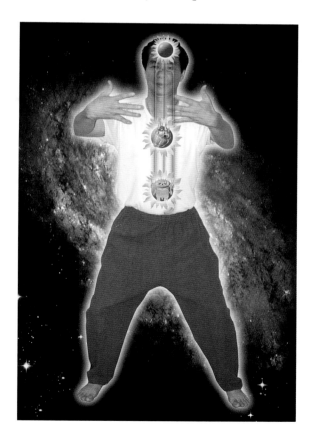

Fig. 5.3. Mind, body, and spirit are all connected.

deal with each one separately. However, those parts affect each other. An approach that does not take that interaction into account ends up with unanticipated side effects in the connected areas. People who have serious physical accidents often have serious emotional aftereffects, for example. Another example would be that people who have had multiple traumas in childhood tend to have chronic pain as well. People who have addictions are affected physically, emotionally, mentally, and spiritually by their affliction. Not working with all of the levels and how they interact with each other often leaves people with unresolved accumulations of toxic energy in various levels of their functioning.

Separating East from West

Eastern and Western beliefs about health and healing seem to operate in conflicting and opposite ways. The West focuses on the concrete aspects of reality, the parts that we can detect with our senses. The East

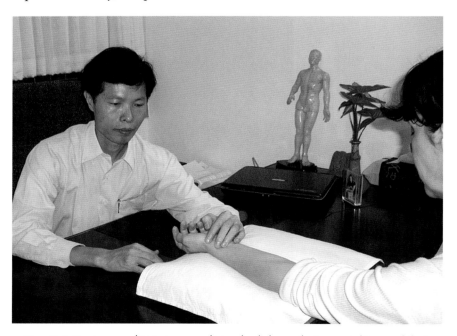

Fig. 5.4. Eastern and Western medicine both have their specialties and their successes. We need to create cooperation between them rather than encourage discrimination against either of them.

tends to emphasize the energetic aspects of reality. However, both of those approaches have legitimacy. It makes more sense to sort out when and how to apply each approach and how they can work together than to try to reject one of the two. Without that recognition, though, many people only make use of the knowledge from one of the systems, even after it seems to have reached the limits of its ability to help them. This can leave them feeling despair if the problems they have developed are serious enough, and it can lead people to extreme and desperate measures.

Overemphasizing Quantitative Research

If someone is offered a new perspective or a new solution about a problem, a common response is "Where is the research to back this up?" The kind of research that they are referring to at those times tends to be quantitative research, the kind in which the problem has been studied in controlled laboratory conditions and particular parts of it have been isolated or manipulated in order to test a particular theory or belief. That type of research certainly has value and has produced many important findings over the years. It is not the only kind of research, however. Learning from the descriptive feedback from individuals in qualitative research, single case studies, and systematic observation has value, too.

The different kinds of research can serve as reality checks for each other. It is important to remember that quantitative research is not completely objective. No research can be completely objective. Research is always based on assumptions. We know that the expectations of the researcher can affect the outcomes of the research, no matter how many controls are put in place. Creating artificial situations and controlled conditions may not lead to results that apply to real situations. Statistics can be manipulated to the point where they completely change the conclusions of a study. As a result many research findings conflict with each other.

We need to pay attention to more than just the results of quantitative research to know what is best for our health and our lives. If we only rely on what current research methods have discovered, we miss out on thousands of years of investigation and learning. Those who rely solely on a reductionistic approach to understanding reality and choose to use quantitative research as their sole guidance for dealing with life are likely to end up feeling confused and frustrated at some point. That type of feeling can eventually lead people to turn to unhealthy options to address their feelings.

INEFFECTIVE SOLUTIONS

Our most common methods of treatment operate in ways that are consistent with the prevailing modes of thought about depression, anxiety, trauma, and addictions. That leads to ineffective solutions.

Narcissists Can Thrive

In a world that celebrates striving and materialism, it makes sense that we also seem to accommodate people whose lifestyle reflects that system. Being narcissistic, driven, greedy, and deceitful is not necessarily celebrated, but it at least seems to be tolerated and overlooked, especially if the people acting that way are considered successful by modern materialistic standards. That can be a source of frustration and resentment, leading to feelings of depression and being overwhelmed in people who are not so egotistical or ruthless, especially if the narcissist is in charge of the solutions.

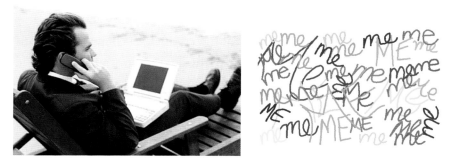

Fig. 5.5. People who reflect the materialistic and "me, me, me" aspects of modern society seem to profit from that attitude.

Government Systems Profit from Pain

The need for many government services is fueled by the problems that are created by the desires and unhappiness of the citizenry. People need licenses to drive and get married. They need doctors and social services to address their ailments, injuries, addictions, relationship and family strife, traumas, and mood disorders. The lifestyles that have created rampant problems may not have come from government services, but the frustration that people experience as a result of receiving unsatisfying, confusing, tedious, or ineffective assistance from those government services, as well as the knowledge that they are paying taxes to keep them running, can be another level of emotional baggage that can lead them to feel depressed, anxious, or overwhelmed.

The reason people are starving is because the
government taxes too much.
This is the reason for starvation.
The reason people are hard to govern is because
their leaders are actively engaged.
This is why they are hard to govern.
The reason people are not serious about death is
because they seek the burdens of life.
This is why they are not serious about death.
Only those who are not slaves to life are wise to
the value of life.

(TAO TE CHING, CHAPTER 77)

Too Much Focus on Diagnosis

Many of our modern methods of healing involve a thorough and detailed assessment and diagnosis of the problem prior to any treatment. In theory that makes sense, but in practice it often creates so many hoops for people to go through in order to get help that they either give up trying at some point or their symptoms get worse while

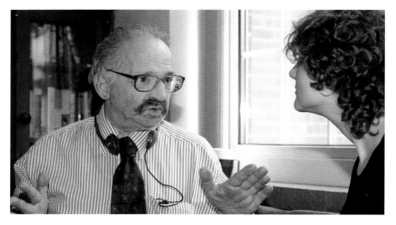

Fig. 5.6. Diagnosis is an important aspect of assessment
but is not a substitute for treatment.

they are going through the process. Teaching people how to be healthy seems important, and yet it is not systematically offered on a widespread basis.

Solutions Are Part of the Problem

Linear solutions are often limited in their effectiveness when trying to solve problems that involve multiple layers of cycles and paradox. In fact, they often make the presenting problems worse. Linear solutions involve breaking the problem into component parts and then addressing the symptoms of each component with a separate solution or set of solutions. Each solution, like any other aspect of nature, will have pros and cons. Everything in life has an upside and a downside. Side effects are a downside of medications, for example. A single problem might be divided into several subproblems, each with its own attempted solutions that have their own downsides. As a result the solutions to a single problem create new problems. One obvious example of that might be how we have used technology to try to save time only to find we have to work more to be able to buy the latest gadgets and learn more so we can know how to use them. Another example might be the bureaucracy that is involved in getting service from a government department.

Our lack of understanding of the cyclical nature of life has led us to create formulas and patterns that have become a new cycle that prevents us from seeing the other ones. We need to learn from Lao Tzu (chapter 36 of the Tao Te Ching):

> *When you want to constrict something,*
> *You must first let it expand;*
> *When you want to weaken something,*
> *You must first enable it;*
> *When you want to eliminate something,*
> *You must first allow it;*
> *When you want to conquer something,*
> *You must first let it be.*
> *This is called the Fine Light.*
> *The weak overcomes the strong;*
> *Fish cannot live away from the source.*
> *The sharp weapon of the nation should never*
> *   be displayed.*

Dissecting nature is useful but putting it back together again in our theories so that the whole of the experience is accounted for is also important. Otherwise our solutions will reflect the problems that are inherent in the situations that we are trying to solve. Imagine trying to use a formula to find your soul mate, for example.

Many Solutions Are Confusing and Not Enjoyable

Many experts from the linear system have their own technical jargon to explain what the problems are and how to solve them. Unless their clients or patients have the same training, they are not likely to understand what they need and how the treatment will help them. Confusing language has taken treatment out of the hands of the common public.

Treatment solutions often involve treatments that taste bad, hurt

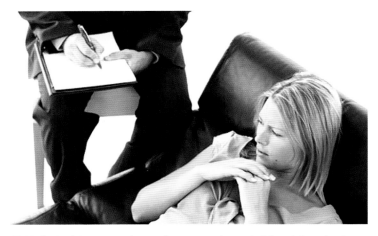

Fig. 5.7. Technical jargon only confuses people and risks giving the impression that they do not know what is good for them.

a lot, or involve drugs with side effects. The treatments are offered in environments that seem sterile and depressing. No wonder they are often not accepted well by the body-mind system.

Most Current Solutions Are Not Sufficient to Resolve Chronic Problems

Conditions like depression, anxiety, addictions, cancer, and chronic pain have not often been successfully resolved with modern approaches. They all seem to develop from more than one factor and affect more than one level of functioning. However, not all of those factors are treated with modern methods. The accumulation of toxins is not addressed, nor is the trauma to the tissues after surgery, for example. Since physical problems can be partially created or made worse by the psychological functioning of the afflicted people, it is not surprising that reductionist approaches that only address the physical symptoms have not yet been able to find a way to reliably cure such conditions.

Too many treatments are focused on the symptoms rather than the source of the problem. A treatment approach that requires a per-

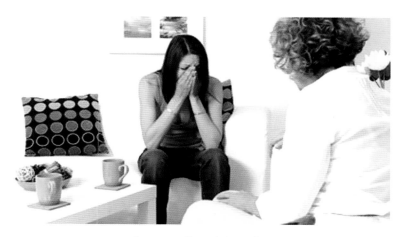

Fig. 5.8. Solutions will work best if they do not
overwhelm the person in the process.

son to treat each symptom or area of functioning separately requires
a lot of time, effort, and money. Imagine the number of professionals
and approaches that would need to be employed to respond to all the
related aspects of a human being.

A LACK OF ENLIGHTENED AND
INFORMED SUPPORT

Loved ones naturally have trouble understanding how people become
traumatized or addicted. They are not aware of all the factors that are
involved. They are also conditioned to believe that the current system
works as well as it could. As a result, instead of questioning and changing the aspects of the system that contribute to the problems that their
loved ones have, they end up judging the people suffering from their
adverse effects. At the same time, the people they are trying to help
seem resistant to getting better. Trying to offer concrete solutions to
someone who is depressed, traumatized, or addicted is not that easy,
even when our hearts are full of compassion.

Many conditions are not easily remedied with logic. It would be

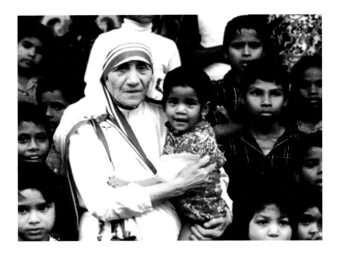

Fig. 5.9. Solutions need to come from a place of understanding and compassion.

nice if people could just "smarten up," "grow up," "lighten up," or "wake up," but all the weight of past and present dynamics are weighing them down. Feeling misunderstood and judged by others often adds to the shame that traumatized and addicted people feel. They feel flawed on some level and often develop deep-seated beliefs that they are somehow not as good or worthy as everyone else. That can make it difficult to believe that they can change and, of course, difficult to take action to find out that they can.

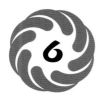

Combining EMDR with Chi Kung

A New Holistic Approach to Solving Emotional Problems

The previous chapters have provided us with a sobering picture of how negative cycles can create blockages in our energetic systems, resulting in a dark, cloudy, slow, thick, and stagnant flow of energy that blocks the free flow of energy we need to feel well and full of life. If this is happening to you, you end up feeling tired, sore, depressed, anxious, and lacking in some vague way. Your gut instinct ends up being full of knots and tangles. How can we prevent this? How can you heal from such a complex tangle of problems on so many levels of your functioning?

Here we offer you a new self-healing approach that takes into account the cycles and energetic pileup that can occur. The new approach provides you with concrete, step-by-step instruction on how to tap into your natural healing mechanisms to clear out and transform blockages in your energetic pathways and take charge of your well-being. This new approach—which we call "Taoist Emotional Recycling"— arises from a combination of EMDR, Eye Movement Desensitization and Reprocessing, with the Universal Healing Tao system of Chi Kung principles and practices.

Integrating elements of the EMDR protocol into the Universal Healing Tao Chi Kung system allows for some important fine-tuning of the technique. The new approach provides more emphasis on the body and a more systematic way of thoroughly processing the pileup of emotional baggage that is stored in the rivers and streams of the body. The approach is clearly and formally integrated into the existing system of knowledge that comprises the Universal Healing Tao.

This integration and synthesis allows practitioners to have more of an understanding of how EMDR works and how continued use of the approach in combination with other healthy routines can create a lasting sense of well-being. As part of a healthy lifestyle, the new approach can be used individually as a form of self-healing. It is suitable for both prevention and treatment. It can also be used by practitioners as a treatment method for their clients. In contrast to modern competitive and materialistic society, the Universal Healing Tao Chi Kung system teaches people how to live in harmony with nature rather than try to conquer it. Working with the vital energies of the body provides viable ways to resolve the seemingly irreconcilable issues and destructive cycles inside of us.

THE EMDR APPROACH

There are steps and phases in the EMDR protocol. First the counselor explains how EMDR works, what the person will be required to do, and what will happen in the process. Then the client is exposed to the different kinds of bilateral processing as a basis for choosing which method she or he prefers. Then the client is led through two preliminary exercises, which provide an experiential sample of what EMDR does and prepare the client for the more difficult work ahead.

Then the therapist asks eight specific questions about the issue that the client has chosen to address. The client's responses to those questions provide the information that is needed to set up the three treatment phases that follow.

1. The first treatment phase is the Desensitization Phase. That is where the negative feelings or urges in connection to a specific issue that the client has chosen to address are processed away.

2. The second treatment phase is called the Positive Installation Phase. That involves building up the positive beliefs that the client wants to have in connection to the issue.

3. The third and final phase of the EMDR treatment process is called the Body Scan. In that phase the focus is on removing any tension, pain, or odd physical feelings that still remain after the first two phases are completed.

THE UNIVERSAL HEALING TAO

Good Food, Good Water, Good Heart, Good Mind,
Good Intentions

TAO GARDEN, THAILAND

The Universal Healing Tao Chi Kung system is an integrated set of the ancient Taoist practices. These practices used to be reserved for people from the East, but they are now being shared with the Western world. At a time in human history in which we have the power to destroy our planet, it is more important than ever for us to share our knowledge of healing as far and wide as possible. In the Universal Healing Tao there are some practices that are meant to be performed while sitting down, others that are performed while standing, some practices that involve standing and moving, and others that are performed while lying on the ground. Unlike many other systems, the Universal Healing Tao embraces the powerful and sacred nature of our sexual energy and teaches us how to use that energy for our health and sense of well-being.

The Universal Healing Tao provides practices that people can use to create a healthy lifestyle. The practices teach people how to manage themselves rather than rely on a government system or other external forces. Relaxation and concentration training are built into the exercises. Doing Chi Kung makes people feel good, so the motivation to continue to practice and become more relaxed and focused is built-in as well. The practices do not require a person to retreat from or reject modern society. The practices go with the person.

The Universal Healing Tao practices teach people how to balance, strengthen, and detoxify themselves on all levels and thereby create an internal flow of energy that can increase the person's chances of good fortune. When it comes to energy, like attracts like. Cultivating positive energy within us invites positive energy into our lives. Practicing regularly leads to greater self-awareness and self-discipline. There are automatic improvements in the ability to concentrate and to relax.

Taoism is a philosophical system that does not require anyone to abandon his or her belief system or to adopt a new one. The Universal Healing Tao applies Taoist concepts in practices that create balanced and healthy energy within us. The concepts within the practices are easy enough to understand. Energy is one language to which we can all relate. People often refer to the state of their own energy or the energy they felt from another person or group of people. A person might say, "I feel drained" or "That speech was electrifying," "That guy gives off bad vibes," or "You could cut the tension in there with a knife." In short, the Universal Healing Tao provides a comprehensive and integrated system of principles and practices that can provide seekers of health and healing with the answers they seek. The practices contained in the system provide people with tools to connect with the source of their knowledge and existence and pathways that lead them back to that source as they live in this world and after their physical existence ceases.

"You Do It, You Get It"

In contrast to many other psychological approaches and healing practices, the benefits of the Universal Healing Tao practices can be felt by anyone, even if you are skeptical of their validity. The crucial factor to experience the benefits of this type of Chi Kung is not that you believe but that you practice. Over time you will increasingly tune in to the energy within and around you and feel it more strongly in your body.

The practices have been developed and refined for over five thousand years through systematic observation. Current research methods are now verifying the value of working with the vital energy in the body. If you want to read more about that, you could read the book called *The Energy Healing Experiments* by Gary E. Schwartz, Ph.D. In addition, Daniel J. Siegel wrote a book called *The Mindful Brain*, in which he examines the connection between mindfulness and well-being. Another source of such research on the benefits of Chi Kung would be the website www.daoistcenter.org. For more in-depth information on the foundational practices of the Universal Healing Tao system, please refer to the bibliography at the end of this book.

FOUNDATIONAL CONCEPTS OF TAOISM

The concepts in Taoism offer us a way to gain a clearer understanding of how all the aspects of life are connected as well as how to move with them effectively. The aspects of nature are reflected and contained within all levels of reality. The ancient phrase is "As above, so below."

Source

For thousands of years the Taoists have realized that at one time there was nothing (referred to as the "Wu Chi"), which had within it the potential to create everything. As in the big bang theory, there was an explosion and the original potential energy went through countless divisions, starting with dividing into two, which refers to the yin and the yang polarity that divides existence into light versus dark, good versus evil, active versus passive, male versus female, and so on. Then there was a division into three (called the Three Pure Ones). Eventually the five elements of earth, fire, water, metal, and wood were created. Each of the five elements has a corresponding color, taste, smell, sound, direction, season, yin organ, yang organ, sense organ, and planet (see fig. 6.1 on page 96).

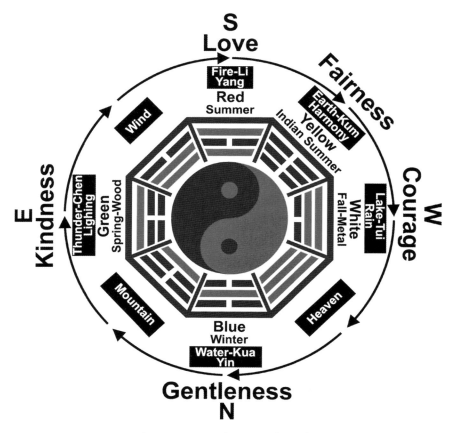

Fig. 6.1. The connections between the colors, sounds, organs, elements, seasons, and forces

This process is described by Lao Tzu in chapter 42 of the Tao Te Ching:

Tao gives rise to one.
One gives rise to two.
Two gives rise to three.
Three gives rise to all things.
All things carry yin and embrace yang.
Drawing Chi together into harmony.
What the world hates is the widow and orphan
  without support.

But lords and rulers name themselves these.
Do not seek gain from losing, or loss from gaining.
What people teach, after discussion becomes
    doctrine.
Those who excel in strength do not prevail after
    death.
I would use this as the father of teaching.

These divisions continued until modern reality was created with all the different sounds, smells, tastes, forces, seasons, personalities, directions, colors, textures, planets, and forces that we experience now (fig. 6.2). As those divisions have continued, some darker and denser

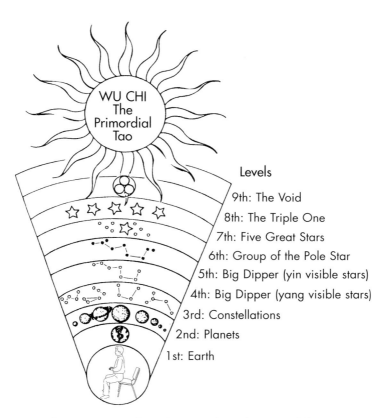

Fig. 6.2. The progression from the Wu Chi to the myriad things

energies have formed, but they are still energy. Everything is energy. Everything vibrates.

Yin and Yang

Most people would recognize the yin/yang symbol from Taoism, but many would not know much about what it represents. Altogether the symbol represents the duality of human experience. We experience life as composed of various pairs of opposites: men and women, adults and children, black and white, active and receptive, positive and negative, hard and soft, and big and small are examples.

But notice in the symbol (fig. 6.3) that there is a tiny dot of white in the black half and a tiny dot of black in the white half. This reminds us that existence is never totally black and white. No situation is totally good or totally bad.

Also of note is the fact that the two halves of the symbol are not divided with a straight line. The curved line reflects the way life operates as we journey in various directions. As we become clearer about one side of existence we can suddenly realize that we are not that far away from the other side anymore. People will often say there is a fine line between genius and insanity, for instance. It is important to remem-

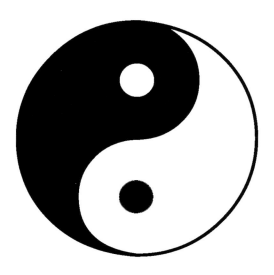

Fig. 6.3. Yin/yang symbol

ber that the line between the two halves also represents the interaction between the two. We often refer to the "chemistry" or "sparks" between people in everyday conversation.

The line between yin and yang reminds us that yin and yang are part of life and necessary to complete the circuit between us and other people and experiences. We cannot understand and appreciate positive experiences without understanding their opposite; the two types of experiences are necessary to complete each other. The dark side is not viewed as a mistake or something to be destroyed. It is accepted as part of the duality of nature and it is accepted that both sides of the duality of nature will always be there. In Taoism we try to make friends with the dark side and create cooperation between the two halves of the whole.

It is also important that the outside rim of the yin/yang symbol is a circle. That points out the continual rolling movement of life. Life never stops. Change is inevitable and continual. The circular shape also reflects the cyclical nature of life. Our interactions with each other and nature are dynamic. All elements of nature respond to each other. Try to sink Rice Krispies in your cereal bowl, give a cat a bath, or catch a butterfly on your finger, and you will see that for yourself.

Going with the Flow

The properties and actions of water are often used to help us understand how to apply Taoist concepts. Water is soft, adaptable, and pliant but cannot be destroyed. It becomes the shape of whatever contains it. No matter what element it is exposed to, it just changes its constitution to suit the environment. For example, if it gets too cold, it becomes ice.

We human beings are approximately two-thirds water. So it makes sense to understand how to move through life like water: to "go with the flow," as in Tao Te Ching, chapter 80:

> *Nothing in the world is softer and more supple*
> *than water.*

When confronting strength and hardness nothing
can overcome it.
Using nothing simplifies.
Using water overcomes hardness.
Using weakness overcomes strength.
There is no one in the world who does not know it,
but no one can apply it.
So it is a saying of sages that:
Whoever can bear the disgrace of the country is the
ruler of the country.
Whoever can bear the misfortune of the world is
the ruler of the world.
Truthful speech seems paradoxical.

Taoism highlights the inherent paradoxes and cycles of nature and points the way to figuring out how to work with them instead of struggling against them. Nature, animals, and children have been closely observed by Taoists for thousands of years to help understand the natural energetic principles of the universe and how to work with them. Animals and children operate in a less self-conscious fashion. They do not question if what they do is "cool" or appropriate. They just naturally do what feels good and works for them. This notion is not exclusive to Taoism. The 12-step community, for example, phrases the goal as "Living life on life's terms."

Just as there are gravitational pulls between the planets and there are currents in rivers that travel down particular paths, people have energetic currents in their bodies that sometimes operate at different points like lakes, rivers, streams, and oceans. Sometimes they get clogged due to tension or toxins in the body. The Universal Healing Tao provides tools that we can use to draw energy from around us and move it smoothly through the natural pathways within us (which are called "meridians"). The divisions within us are dissolved and we feel more grounded, connected, and peaceful inside. We also feel more open and connected to the outside world. Having the experience of smooth, harmonious flow allows us to recognize when we are not operating in a manner consistent with that feeling in dealing with other people and situations outside of us. Then we can take steps to correct our attitudes, beliefs, and actions so that we are not locked in a power struggle with life anymore. The energy within us is lighter as a result, becoming more and more similar to the undivided, pure energy of the Source as we continue to practice.

Dense Energy Becomes Lighter— It's All an Inside Job

We now know that violet light fills the universe. It is more concentrated in certain areas. The North Star provides the largest concentration in our universe (fig. 6.4). Violet light is intelligent. It contains the universal knowledge. It is also programmable.

When we do not have enough love in our hearts we lose our wireless connection with the violet light. Then we lose our connection with the universal knowledge. We need that connection to multiply the good energy inside of us. Without it, we start to lose our way. Our cells

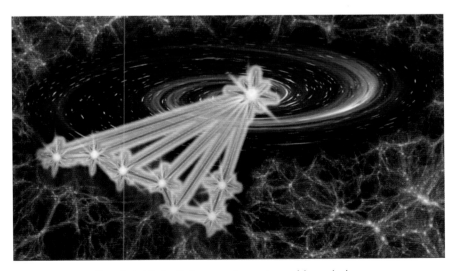

Fig. 6.4. Violet light contains universal knowledge.

cannot be healed properly anymore. That can lead to addiction and cancer. We need to clean our energy systems and maintain the connection with the violet energy to heal and stay healthy (fig. 6.5). We need to transform the sexual energy, our highest vibration, to intelligent, vio-

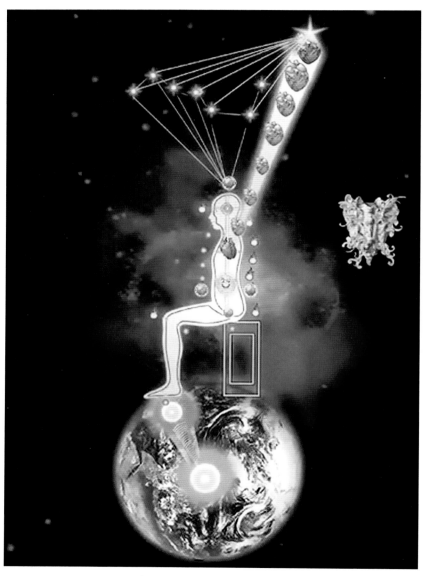

Fig. 6.5. Cleaning our energy systems maintains
our connection with violet energy.

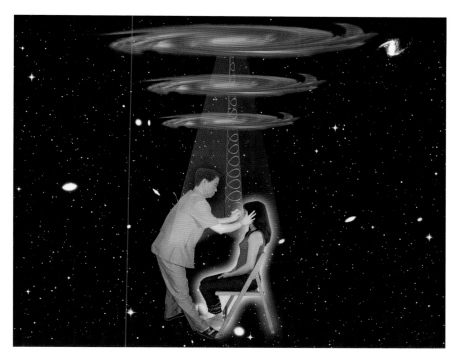

Fig. 6.6. In the Tao we believe that we cannot receive what we want and need until we work to refine our energy and use it to help others.

let soul energy. This includes transforming the dark and cloudy energy that is left over from experiences from the past that we have not be able to accept.

In the Tao we believe that if you transform and refine your energy, create a connection to the violet energy, and give and empty yourself, the universe will fill you up with healing and universal knowledge (fig. 6.6). If you are not clean you cannot receive. You cannot give garbage and receive energy back.

Practitioners learn humility as we are continually reminded through the practices that we are tiny drops swimming in an ocean of chi. Compassion increases as we learn how little the average person knows about how to manage his or her energy and recognize that as long as we are judging or resenting someone else then we have more work to do to master our own energy.

ADVANTAGES OF THE NEW APPROACH

The Universal Healing Tao practices show us ways in which we do not have to fear the negative in life. We can embrace it, transform it, and use it to create new, healthy energy for ourselves. We can welcome the denser and darker energies in our lives and transform them in a way similar to how coal is turned into a diamond. In a sense, the Universal Healing Tao is an ancient recycling program. However, we recycle more than our paper, cardboard, metal, and plastics. We also recycle our toxic emotions. Rather than spewing them into the air with nasty words or letting them fester and rot inside of our minds and bodies, we transform them and send them into the earth to be recycled. Just as we breathe in oxygen and breathe out carbon dioxide and the earth does the opposite, we can send our toxins into the earth and it can transform them into energy that can be given back to us.

Detoxification and balance are not meant to be activities that we do every few years like a tune-up for a car. The more we keep our systems clean, balanced, and strong, the more we can stay in clear contact with the purer and lighter formative energies of the universe and the universal knowledge that surrounds us.

As people practice Chi Kung they tend to expel toxins in a variety of ways, such as sneezing, belching, passing gas, crying, blowing their noses, defecating, urinating, and vomiting. From an energy-based perspective, we do not view this as disgusting or inappropriate (although we do not go out of our way to ignore or defy local cultural traditions). Is it really better to keep all of your toxins inside, rotting away, so you do not expel them and do something that others might consider impolite? If we keep our emotional and environmental toxins inside, they act like rust in the body. We become prematurely weak and old. Wrinkles, gray hair, and aches and pains start to form as the channels that distribute our energy inside become clogged.

The Universal Healing Tao system is systematic and comprehensive in its ability to teach people how to heal themselves, first with an emphasis on the body, then on the emotions, and then eventually focusing more on the spirit. So combining Universal Healing Tao practices with EMDR provides a more complete and effective method for clearing deep-seated emotional problems from your system than practicing EMDR alone.

1. The new approach does not require much explanation in order to prepare the client.

2. Unlike EMDR alone, the unconscious connections to the issue that is being addressed do not often come to mind during the process, but they still get addressed. That often makes the experience less emotional and more able to be done as a self-healing practice.

3. Because the internal organs are the source of mental, emotional, and physical health, focusing more on the body and more particularly on the internal organs allows the effects of the issue to be addressed without identifying and targeting each level separately.

4. People can focus on the issue any way they want instead of coming up with a specific picture from their memories. Not everyone has visual memories connected to the issue that they want to address.

5. The approach can easily be adapted to be used with a group.

6. The building up of positive beliefs—which are needed to address the issue if it comes up again—seems to happen automatically.

7. People do not usually get tired when they do the practice.

8. The approach is simple enough that, after an initial session or two, most people can practice on their own by following a short written summary.

9. Some people who have not been able to do EMDR have had success using this combined practice because there are more built-in aspects to keep them calm throughout the process.

10. Some people feel the charge around their chosen issue to be removed within a few sets of processing.

KEY ELEMENTS OF
TAOIST EMOTIONAL RECYCLING

The following are the essential elements of the practice that can help you release and dissolve the negative feelings about things that have happened in your life that you have been unable to let go of on your own.

Visualization Leads to Actualization

An ancient Chi Kung saying is "Where the mind goes, the chi follows." It is also true that where the chi goes, the blood follows. Chi is not an intelligent energy but it can go anywhere, across tissues, across space, and across time. If we focus our mind and connect with the violet energy we can create healing inside us on all levels.

Tuning In to Our Organs

In our system, in line with Chinese medicine theory, we believe that our mental, physical, emotional, and spiritual health are created in our internal organs. Some of our internal organs are solid. They are called yin organs. They are the transformers for the energy that comes from our food and our surroundings. When they are in balance they produce virtues and health on all levels. When they are out of balance they produce toxins, negative thoughts, negative feelings, and physical deterioration. Each yin organ is paired with a yang organ, a sense organ, a direction, a color, a season, a sound, and an element.

The organs are the transformers that allow us access to those dimensions. They have memory. Our memories are stored in the internal organs. Entire books have been written on that subject. One example is Paul Pearsall's book *The Heart's Code,* which offers fascinating accounts of heart transplant patients who ended up experiencing feelings, preferences, and even memories of the people from whom they received their new hearts. It provides support for the Taoist idea that our health on all levels is produced through and stored in our internal organs.

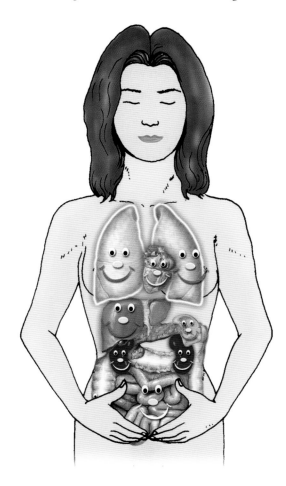

Fig. 6.7. Smiling produces chemical reactions that warm the energy in the body and facilitate the healing process.

Smiling

When we smile, a number of amazing chemical reactions can happen in the body (fig. 6.7). When we smile and focus on a particular internal organ we can direct the benefits of smiling energy to that organ. If we smile to each internal organ in the correct order, known as the "creative cycle," we can transform the toxic energy in each of the organs one at a time, create the virtues in each organ, and combine the virtues in an order in which they complement each other. Altogether those virtues combine to create compassion. Details of the correct order are given in the next chapter in the Inner Smile exercise.

Focusing on Colors

Color is an energy frequency. Focusing on the correct color as you focus on each internal organ will bring the correct frequency of chi to that organ so it can be balanced and healed to its natural healthy state (fig. 6.8).

The correct color to see when you focus on the heart is red.

Seeing a yellow spleen inside you will help you to fine-tune its energy.

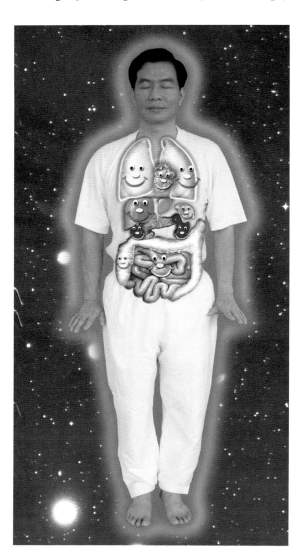

Fig. 6.8. Focusing on the correct color for each organ helps to tune it with the correct frequency of vibration.

White is the correct color to see when focusing on your lungs.

Focusing on the color blue while concentrating on your kidneys will detoxify and energize them.

In order to bring the right kind of chi to your liver you should see the color green around it.

Smile and focus on the correct color for each organ and watch until the color becomes clear and bright around it. When it is dark and cloudy, there are still toxic emotions being produced in that organ. Smiling to each organ in the correct way can transform that toxic energy and cultivate the virtues in it.

Using Eye Movements to Release Stuck Energy

Many traditions have recognized the connection between our eyes and our spirit. A common saying is that the eyes are the windows to the soul. Neuro-linguistic programming (NLP) has recognized that our eyes focus in different directions when we think about the past, present, or future. Traditional Chinese medicine recognizes that the eyes are energetically connected to the whole body and therefore can affect the health of the whole body. Taoism has recognized the power of the eyes to direct chi for thousands of years.

In order to undo the energetic knots and tangles in our systems that have formed due to some or all of the unhealthy contributing factors that were listed earlier, we need to find those unhealthy barriers and use eye movements in a new way to release them. This requires focusing the mind on the right issue, color, and point on the body, and then manually moving the eyes in a way that will dissolve the blockage. As the blockages are dissolved, the access to the universal knowledge from the Source becomes more accessible. Do not be surprised by what you think about, emotionally feel, physically feel, or picture as you go through the process. You are not weird or crazy. In fact, if your experiences during the exercise are unexpected and confusing, that probably means you are doing it right.

Moving your eyes in different ways can help move the energy in your body and produce specific benefits. Moving the eyes in the proper way while you focus on an upsetting experience can help you to complete the processing and transform the emotion around the event into virtuous energy.

- Moving eyes from side to side, looking left and right, can delete the connection to memories from the past. It creates an alternating current of electricity that can break up the energy inside.
- Moving the eyes in spirals into positive thoughts, feelings, and body sensations, while connected to the energy of each solid internal organ, can help you to recycle and transform the emotional energy connected to an issue from the past (fig. 6.9).

  Spiraling out, making spirals that are becoming progressively bigger, brings out the experience (and often intensifies it), while spiraling inward in progressively smaller circles gathers the energy.
- Moving the eyes in a vertical figure-eight pattern helps you connect to the energy of eternity.
- Moving them in a horizontal figure-eight pattern helps you connect to the energy of infinity.
- Rolling the eyes back in a circle helps move energy up the front part of the body (the Functional Channel) and down the back (the Governor or Regulator Channel) to help keep you calm.
- Moving them down the front and up the back helps stimulate energy flow in the other direction, which will help to energize you and increase your focus.

Most of the processing in this technique uses multiples of nine movements. Nine is an important number in Taoism. It is a number of returning. For example, nine times two equals eighteen. One plus eight brings us back to the number nine. Nine times three equals twenty-seven. Two plus seven brings us back to the number nine.

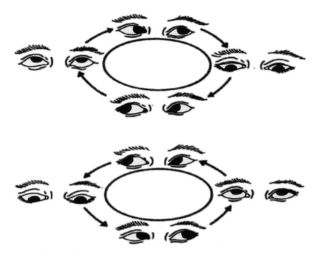

Fig. 6.9. Taoists have been using eye movements for thousands of years to move the energy through people in powerful ways to promote healing.

We can use a computer analogy to guide our understanding of how the energy around a past trauma, trigger, phobia, or pain can be transformed by this method. When you want to remove a file from your computer, you first access that file, then hit the delete key and send it to the recycling bin, then activate the "empty recycle bin" function to activate the recycling and transforming process and create more space. In this practice, back and forth eye movements are used to delete the file and the links to it, and the spiraling and spinning movements are used to recycle and transform the experience and create new, positive energy.

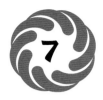

Foundational Taoist Practices for Cleansing the Organs

The Inner Smile, Microcosmic Orbit, and Six Healing Sounds

Our internal organs are the transformers for our physical, mental, emotional, and spiritual health. When we balance, detoxify, and strengthen the chi in the internal organs, we can improve our health and sense of well-being on all levels. Each internal organ can produce certain negative emotions if it is too toxic or out of balance. Each organ can also produce particular virtues if it is clean and in balance.

The heart produces hastiness, impatience, hatred, and cruelty when it is toxic or out of balance. Balancing its energy produces the virtues of joy, happiness, and love. It helps us to feel good about the future.

Our spleen can create worry, negative thinking, and overthinking within us if it is not healthy. When its energy is cleansed and balanced, it can help us feel openness and trust.

When our lungs are in balance they produce the virtues of courage and righteousness. When they are struggling they can create grief, sadness, loss, and depression.

Fear, anxiety, phobias, and trauma are registered in the kidneys when they are toxic. Gentleness, calmness, and stillness are produced when those toxins are removed or transformed. The kidneys are connected to emotions about events from our past. Balance in the kidneys helps to create forgiveness and peace inside about things that have happened in the past.

The liver produces anger, frustration, jealousy, envy, and shame when its energy is out of balance. Generosity and kindness are produced when its energy is balanced.

THE INNER SMILE

The Inner Smile meditation, which draws positive energy to the internal organs and glands, is an ancient Taoist Chi Kung practice that teaches people how to properly restore peace inside them. It initiates the Microcosmic Orbit practice, which provides a healthy circulation of energy through all of the organs. There are two major channels in the body, the Functional Channel and the Governor Channel. The Functional Channel runs more along the front of the body and the Governor Channel is more on the back. The two channels connect to form an elliptical orbit around the body. The points along the orbit connect to the other acupuncture channels in the body.

 ## Inner Smile Meditation

To begin the Inner Smile meditation, sit on the edge of a chair with your hands held together and eyes closed.

Front Line: The Functional Channel

1. Be aware of smiling cosmic energy in front of you and breathe it into your eyes.

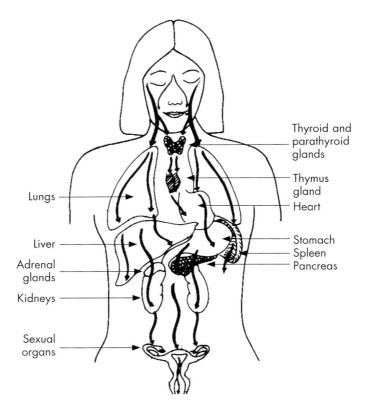

Thyroid and parathyroid glands

Thymus gland

Heart

Lungs

Liver

Adrenal glands

Kidneys

Sexual organs

Stomach

Spleen

Pancreas

Fig. 7.1. Front line smile: major vital organs

2. Allow smiling energy to enter the point between your eyebrows. Let it flow into your nose and cheeks, and let it lift up the corners of your mouth, as you bring your tongue to rest on your palate.
3. Smile down to your neck, throat, thyroid, parathyroid, and thymus.
4. Smile into your heart, feeling joy and love spread out from there to the lungs, liver, spleen, pancreas, kidneys, and genitals (fig. 7.1).

⦿ Middle Line: The Digestive Tract

1. Bring smiling energy into the eyes, then down to the mouth.
2. Swallow saliva as you smile down to your stomach, small intestine (duodenum, jejunum, and ileum), large intestine (ascending

colon, transverse colon, and descending colon), rectum, and anus (fig. 7.2).

⟳ Back Line: The Governor Channel

1. Smile, and look upward about three inches into your mid-eyebrow point and pituitary gland (fig. 7.3).
2. Direct your smile to the Third Room, the small cavity deep in the center of your brain. Feel the room expand and grow with the bright golden light shining through the brain.
3. Smile into the thalamus, pineal gland (Crystal Palace), and the left and right sides of the brain.
4. Smile to the midbrain and the brain stem, then to the base of your skull.

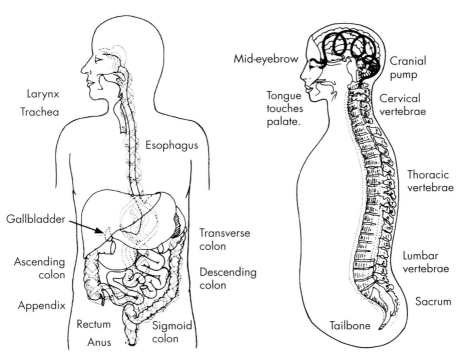

Fig. 7.2. Middle line smile: digestive tract

Fig. 7.3. Back line smile: Governor Channel

5. Smile down to the seven cervical vertebrae, the twelve thoracic vertebrae, the five lumbar vertebrae, then the sacrum and the tailbone.

6. Refresh the loving, soothing smile energy in your eyes, then smile down the front, middle, and back lines in succession. Now do all of them at once, feeling bathed in a cooling waterfall or glowing sunshine of cosmic energy, smiles, joy, and love.

⟳ Collect Energy in the Navel

1. Gather all the smiling energy in your navel area—about 1.5 inches inside your body. Spiral that energy with your mind or your hands from the center point to the outside. (Don't go above the diaphragm or below the pubic bone.)

2. **Men:** Cover your navel with both palms, left hand over right. Collect and mentally spiral the energy outward from the navel 36 times clockwise, and then inward 24 times counterclockwise.

   Women: Cover your navel with both palms, right hand over left. Collect and mentally spiral the energy outward from the navel 36 times counterclockwise, and then inward 24 times clockwise.

3. Finish by storing energy safely in the navel.

THE MICROCOSMIC ORBIT

The Microcosmic Orbit is the foundation of Chi Kung practices. Dedicated practice of this ancient esoteric method eliminates stress and nervous tension, energizes the internal organs, restores health to damaged tissue, and builds a strong sense of personal well-being. The Microcosmic Orbit meditation strengthens the Original Chi and teaches you the basics of circulating chi. It allows the palms, the soles of the feet, the mid-eyebrow point, and the crown point to open. These specific locations are the major points where energy can be absorbed, condensed, and transformed into fresh new life force.

The Microcosmic Orbit meditation awakens, circulates, and directs

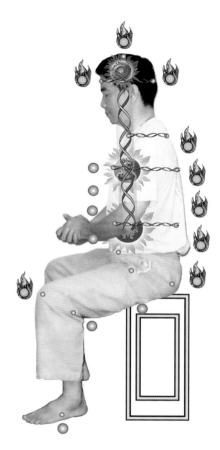

Fig. 7.4. Microcosmic Orbit

chi through the Governor Channel, which ascends up the back of the body from the coccyx (tailbone) to the head, then down the front to the space between the bottom of the nose and the upper lip, and the Functional Channel (or Conception Vessel), which runs up the front of the body from the perineum to the space between the chin and the lower lip (fig. 7.4).

Opening the points along the Microcosmic Orbit and circulating energy through it will provide energy and focus if you circulate it up the back and down the front of the body. It will provide relaxation if you circulate the energy in the opposite direction, up the front and down the back. We use the Microcosmic Orbit in this practice to help you feel balanced.

Microcosmic Orbit Meditation

1. Focus on the lower tan tien (the area where the Original Chi is stored, between the navel, kidneys, and sexual organs). Feel the pulsing in this area, observe whether this area feels tense or relaxed, cool or warm, expansive or contracting. Notice any sensations of chi: tingling, heat, expansiveness, pulsing, electric, or magnetic sensations. Allow these to grow and expand. Then let this energy flow out to the navel center.

2. Use your intention (mind-eye-heart power) to spiral in the navel point, guiding and moving the chi. Let the energy flow down to the sexual center (Ovarian or Sperm Palace, both located at the pubic bone).

3. Move the energy from the sexual center to the perineum and down to the soles of the feet.

4. Draw the energy up from the soles to the perineum and to the sacrum.

5. Draw the energy up from the sacrum to the Door of Life (the point in the spine opposite the navel).

6. Draw the energy up to the mid-spine point (the T11 vertebra).

7. Draw the energy up to the base of the skull (Jade Pillow).

8. Draw the energy up to the crown.

9. Move the energy down from the crown to the mid-eyebrow point.

10. Touch the tip of your tongue to your upper palate, press and release a few times; then lightly touch the palate, sensing the electric or tingling feeling in the tip of the tongue. Move the energy down from the mid-eyebrow to where the tip of your tongue and palate meet.

11. Move the energy down from the palate through your tongue to the throat center.

12. Move the energy down from the throat to the heart center.

13. Bring the energy down from the heart to the solar plexus and feel a small sun shining out.

14. Bring the energy back down to the navel.

15. Continue to circulate your energy through this entire sequence of points, at least 9 times. Once the pathways are open, you can let your energy flow continuously like a river of energy without needing to stop at each point.

16. Conclude when you wish by collecting energy at the navel (see specific directions for men and women on page 116 at the end of the Inner Smile meditation).

For more details on this practice see Mantak Chia's *Healing Light of the Tao*.

SIX HEALING SOUNDS

Each of your internal organs can be cooled and detoxified further using a specific sound. You can use those sounds to help yourself keep as calm as possible as you are working through whatever issue you choose to address. In the sound exercises below you can do the sounds without the hand movements. However, if you have already received training in the full Six Healing Sounds meditation you can do the hand movements if you like.

The Lungs' Sound: First Cosmic Healing Sound

The lungs' sound is a metal sound. It sounds like the vibration of a bell and activates the lung chi.

Characteristics

Associated Organ: Large intestine
Element: Metal
Season: Autumn

Color: White

Emotions: Grief and sadness

Virtues: Courage and righteousness

Related Senses: Smell (nose) and touch (skin)

Taste: Pungent

Related parts of the body: Chest, inner arms, thumbs

Sound: Sss-s-s-s-s-s (tongue behind teeth) (fig. 7.5)

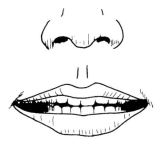

Fig. 7.5. Mouth position for the lungs' sound. Close the jaws so that the teeth meet. Draw the corners of the mouth back.

❂ *Position and Practice*

1. Sit with your back straight, your hands resting on your lungs, and your eyes closed. Smile down to your lungs. Be aware of the quality of the energy in the lungs (fig. 7.6). Picture a white light, fresh and pure like the energy of the mountains, and hear the metal sound.

2. Take a deep breath, open the eyes, and raise your arms out in front of you with the palms facing the lungs (fig. 7.7). When the hands are at eye level, begin to rotate the palms, bringing them above your head until they face up and are pushing outward. Point the fingers toward those of the opposite hand. Keep the elbows rounded out to the sides, and do not straighten your arms (fig. 7.8).

   Close the jaws so that the teeth gently meet and part the lips slightly as you slowly exhale through your teeth the sound "sss-s-s-s-s." In the beginning, you can produce the lungs' sound out loud, but eventually you should practice it subvocally. Feel that the sound starts to move the chi in the lungs, and that any excess heat and toxins are expelled from the lungs as the sacs surrounding the lungs are compressed.

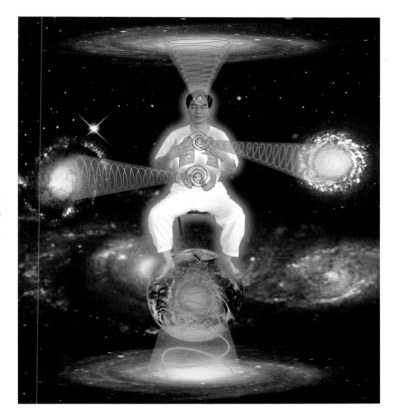

Fig. 7.6. Become aware of the lungs.

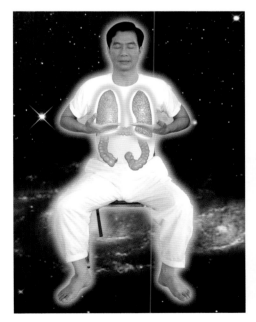

Fig. 7.7. Gather the energy into the lungs.

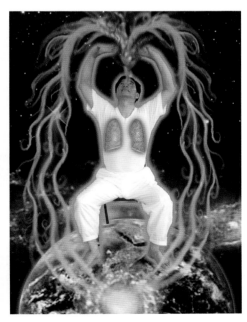

Fig. 7.8. Do the lungs' sound.

Note: *Subvocally* means that you are vocalizing so softly that only you can hear the sound and feel the vibration inside the lungs. You must exhale slowly and fully. Also, the word *sacs* refers to the layers of tissue called fasciae that surround every organ.

3. When you have exhaled completely, rotate the palms and scoop up the white light. Pour this light from the crown down into the lungs (fig. 7.9). Lower the arms and hold your hands before the lungs and radiate the bright white light and courage into the lungs.

4. Rest, close your eyes, and be aware of your lungs. Smile into them,

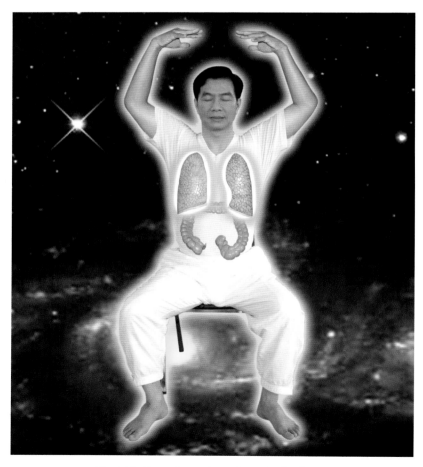

Fig. 7.9. Pour the energy down to the lungs.

and imagine that you are still making the lungs' sound. Feel the vibration of the sound moving and cleaning the energy in the lungs (fig. 7.10). Breathe normally, and see your lungs glowing with a bright white light. This will strengthen your lungs and activate courage in the lungs. With each breath, try to feel that fresh white metal energy is replacing the excess hot, toxic, and depressed energy.

5. Nurture good emotions. This is the most important part of this practice. Take as much time as you need to get in touch with the organs. When you get rid of the excess heat and let the white metal energy expand in the lungs, good emotional qualities will have room to grow. Concentrate on the feelings of righteousness and courage as

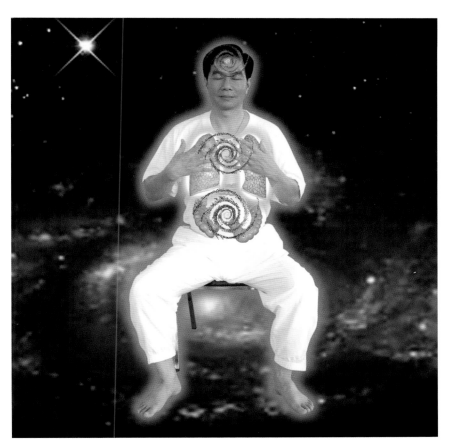

Fig. 7.10. Smile to your lungs.

you transform any sadness or grief. Sit up straight and tall so you can feel courage, and try to maintain the feeling of the lungs' sound for increasingly longer periods after each practice, and in your daily life.

Repeat the lungs' sound 3 to 6 times. For sadness, depression, colds, flu, toothaches, asthma, emphysema, or depression, you may repeat this exercise 6, 9, 12, or 24 times.

The Kidneys' Sound: Second Cosmic Healing Sound

The kidneys' sound is a water sound and it activates the kidney chi.

Characteristics

Associated Organ: Bladder
Element: Water
Season: Winter
Color: Dark blue
Emotion: Fear
Virtue: Gentleness, calmness and stillness, alertness
Parts of the body: Sides of the feet, inner legs, chest
Senses: Hearing (ears), bones
Taste: Salty
Sound: Choo-oo-oo-oo (as when blowing out a candle: lips forming an "O") (fig. 7.11)

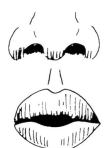

Fig. 7.11. Round the lips, making the sound one makes when blowing out a candle.

◎ *Position and Practice*

1. Sit with your back straight, your hands resting on your kidneys, and your eyes closed. Smile down to your kidneys. Be aware of the quality of the energy in the kidneys. Picture a blue light, the sun shining on the ocean (fig. 7.12).

2. Take a deep breath, open the eyes, and put your legs together, ankles and knees touching. Lean forward and clasp the fingers of both hands together around your knees. Pull your arms straight from the lower back while bending the torso forward (this allows your back

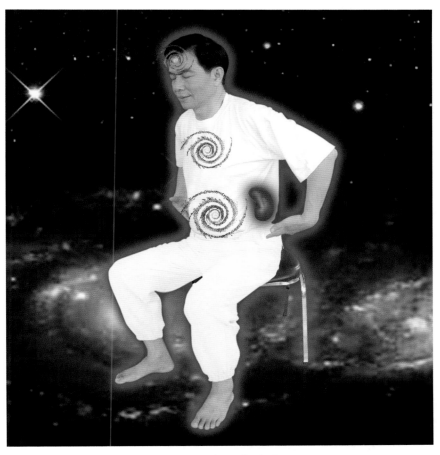

Fig. 7.12. Smile to the kidneys.

to protrude in the area of the kidneys). Simultaneously tilt your head up as you look straight ahead, maintaining the pull on your arms from the lower back. Feel the pull on your spine. Round the lips, and slightly exhale with the sound "choo-oo-oo-oo" as if you were blowing out a candle (fig. 7.13).

Simultaneously contract your abdomen, pulling it in toward your kidneys. At first you can produce the kidneys' sound out loud, but eventually you should practice it subvocally. Feel that the sound starts to move the chi in the kidneys; any excess heat and toxins are expelled from the kidneys as the sacs surrounding the kidneys are compressed.

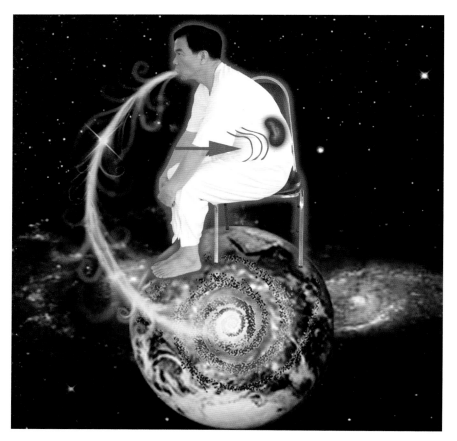

Fig. 7.13. Do the kidneys' sound.

3. After you have fully exhaled, sit erect, separate the legs, and move your arms up to the crown and scoop up the blue light. Pour this light over the body and into the kidneys. Lower your arms and hold the palms on the kidneys. Radiate the blue light, gentleness, and stillness into the kidneys.

4. Return your hands to your kidneys. Rest, close your eyes, and be aware of your kidneys. Listen to your kidneys. Smile to them, and imagine that you are still making the kidneys' sound. Feel the vibration of the sound is moving and cleaning the energy in the kidneys (fig. 7.14).

   Breathe normally, and see your kidneys glowing with a cool blue

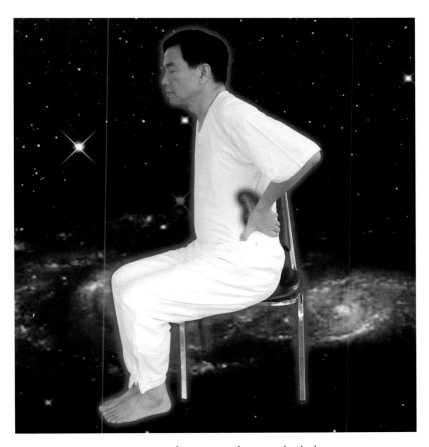

Fig. 7.14. Bring the energy down to the kidneys.

light. This will strengthen your kidneys and activate the gentleness and stillness in the kidneys. With each breath, try to feel that bright blue water energy is replacing the excess hot, toxic, and fear energy (fig. 7.15).

5. Nurture good emotions. This is the most important part of this practice. Take as much time as you need to get in touch with the kidneys. When you get rid of the excess heat and let the cool blue water energy expand in the kidneys, good emotional qualities will have room to grow.

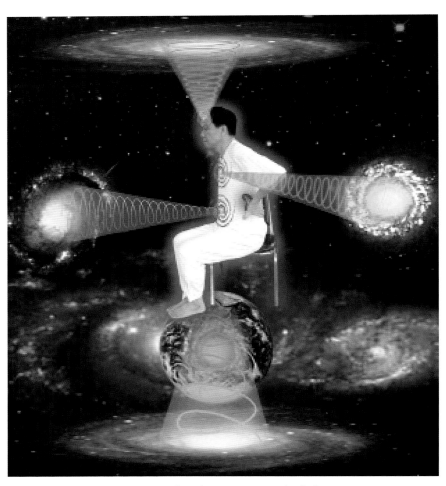

Fig. 7.15. Gather the energy into the kidneys.

Concentrate on the feelings of gentleness, stillness, and alertness as you transform any fear. Feel the gentleness also relaxing the lower back. Try to maintain the sensation of this energy for increasingly longer periods after each practice, and in your daily life.

Repeat the steps from 3 to 6 times. You may repeat this exercise more times to alleviate fear, fatigue, dizziness, ringing in the ears, or back pain.

 ## The Liver's Sound: Third Cosmic Healing Sound

The liver's sound is a wood sound and it activates the liver's chi.

Characteristics

Associated Organ: Gallbladder
Element: Wood
Season: Spring
Color: Green
Emotion: Anger
Virtue: Kindness
Parts of the body: Inner legs, groin, diaphragm, ribs
Senses: Sight (eyes), tears
Taste: Sour
Sound: Sh-h-h-h-h-h-h (tongue near palate) (fig. 7.16)

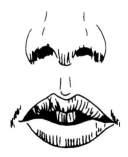

Fig. 7.16. To make the "sh-h-h-h-h-h-h" sound, exhale with the tongue near the palate.

🌀 Position and Practice

1. Sit comfortably with your back straight, your hands resting on your liver, and your eyes closed. Smile down to your liver until you feel you are in touch with your liver (fig. 7.17). Be aware of the quality of the energy in the liver. Picture a forest, a big green forest. See the sun shining on the forest creating life force and green light.

2. Take a deep breath, open the eyes, and extend your arms out to your sides, palms up. Slowly raise the arms from the sides to the crown, following this action with your eyes. Intertwine the fingers, and

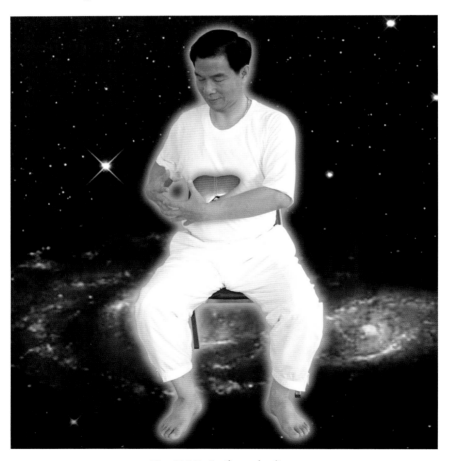

Fig. 7.17. Smile to the liver.

rotate your joined hands to face the ceiling, palms up. Push up and out with the heels of the hands and stretch the arms out from the shoulders; the elbows should be pushing to the back.

Bend slightly to the left, exerting a gentle pull on the liver. Open your eyes wider because they are the openings of the liver. Slowly exhale the sound "sh-h-h-h-h-h-h" out loud and eventually subvocally (fig. 7.18). Feel the sound start to move the energy in the liver, and feel that all excess heat and toxins are expelled from the liver as the sac around it is compressed.

3. After you have fully exhaled, sit erect, separate the hands, and scoop

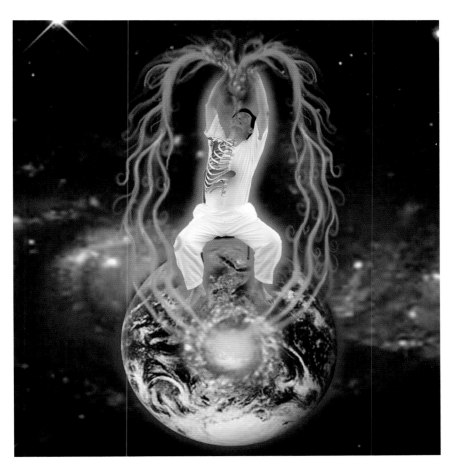

Fig. 7.18. Do the liver's sound.

up the green light. Pour this light over the body and into the liver (fig. 7.19). Slowly bring your arms down, palms facing out, and scoop up more green light and hold both hands before your liver. Radiate the green light, the forest energy, and kindness in the liver.

4. Return your hands to your liver. Rest. Close your eyes and be aware of your liver. Smile and look in your liver and imagine that you are still making the liver's sound. Feel the vibration of the sound moving and cleaning the energy in the liver (fig. 7.20).

Breathe normally, and see your liver glowing with the green

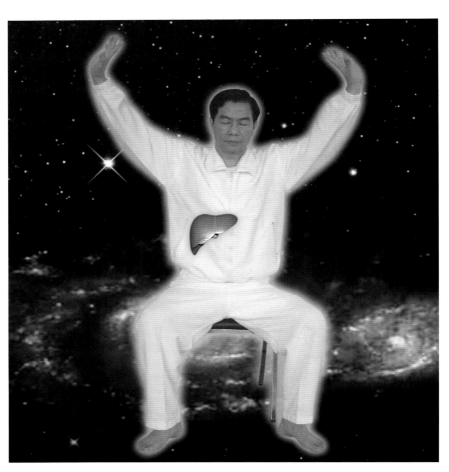

Fig. 7.19. Scoop green light and pour it into the liver.

rejuvenating light. This will strengthen your liver and activate kindness in the liver. With each breath, try to feel that bright green wood energy is replacing the excess hot, toxic, angry aggression and frustration energy.

5. Nurture good emotions. This is the most important part of this practice. Take as much time as you need to get in touch with the liver. When you get rid of the excess heat and let the warm, moist, green wood energy expand in the liver, kindness will have room to grow. Concentrate on the virtues of kindness and forgiveness as you transform any anger and aggression. Feel warm

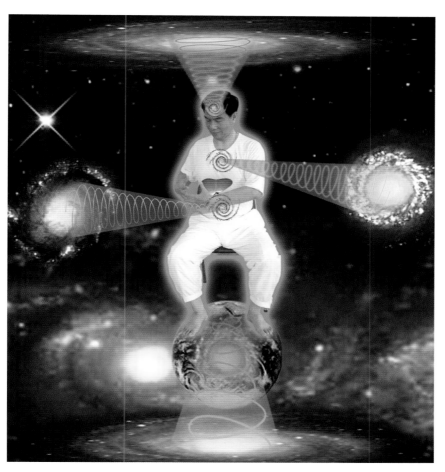

Fig. 7.20. Gather energy into the liver.

and energetic, and maintain this feeling for as long as you can after practice.

Repeat the steps from 3 to 6 times. Practice more to expel anger, to clear red or watery eyes, to remove a sour or bitter taste, and to detoxify the liver.

The Heart's Sound: Fourth Cosmic Healing Sound

The heart's sound is the fire sound and activates the heart energy.

Characteristics

Associated Organ: Small intestine
Element: Fire
Season: Summer
Color: Red
Emotions: Hastiness, arrogance, cruelty
Virtues: Joy, honor, sincerity
Parts of the body: Armpits, inner arms
Senses: Tongue, speech
Taste: Bitter
Sound: Haw-w-w-w-w-w (mouth wide open) (fig. 7.21)

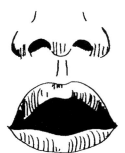

Fig. 7.21. "Haw-w-w-w-w" sound

◉ Position and Practice

1. Sit comfortably with your back straight, your hands resting on your heart, and your eyes closed. Smile down to your heart until you feel you are in touch with your heart (fig. 7.22). Be aware of the quality of the energy in the heart. Picture a sunset on the ocean, a red light.

2. Take a deep breath, open the eyes, and take the same position as for the liver's sound. Unlike the former exercise, however, you will lean slightly to the right to pull gently against the heart, which is located just left of the center of your chest.

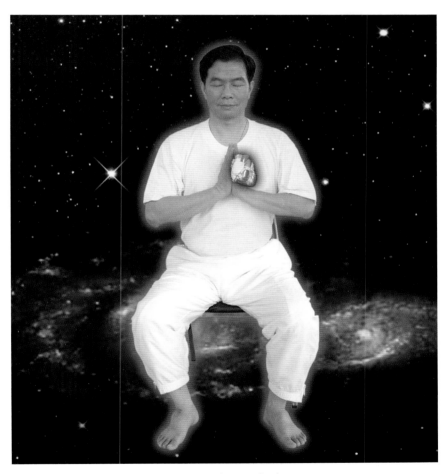

Fig. 7.22. Smile into the heart.

Focus on your heart, feel the tongue's connection to the open mouth, round the lips, and slowly exhale the sound "haw-w-w-w-w-w" out loud and eventually subvocally. Feel the sound start to move the energy in the heart, and feel that excess heat and toxins are expelled from the heart as the sac around it is compressed (fig. 7.23).

3. After you have fully exhaled, sit erect, separate the hands, and scoop up the red light. Pour this light over the body and into the heart

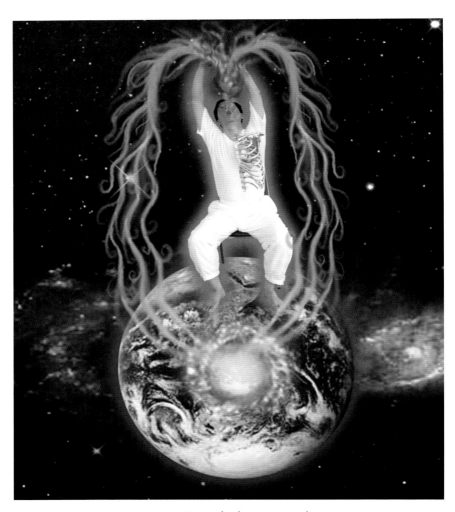

Fig. 7.23. Do the heart's sound.

(fig. 7.24). Slowly bring your arms down, palms facing out. Scoop up more red light and hold both hands before your heart. Radiate the red light, the love, and inner joy into your heart.

4. Return your hands to your heart. Rest, close your eyes, and be aware of your heart. Smile to your heart and imagine that you are still making the heart's sound. Feel the vibration of the sound moving and cleaning the energy in the heart. Breathe normally, and see your heart glowing with a red fire light.

This will strengthen your heart and activate love, inner joy, and

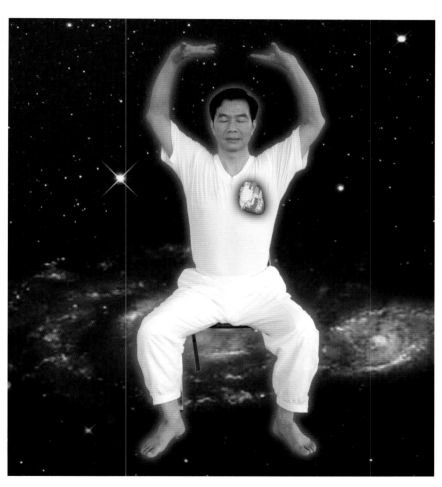

Fig. 7.24. Gather energy into the heart.

sincerity in your heart. With each breath, try to feel that the warm red light is replacing the excess hot, toxic energy and any hastiness, arrogance, and hate in the heart (fig. 7.25).

5. Nurture good emotions. This is the most important part of this practice. Take as much time as you need to get in touch with the heart (fig. 7.26).

When you get rid of the excess heat and let the red fire energy expand in the heart, good emotional qualities will have room to grow. Feel love, joy, honor, and respect radiate outward (fig. 7.27).

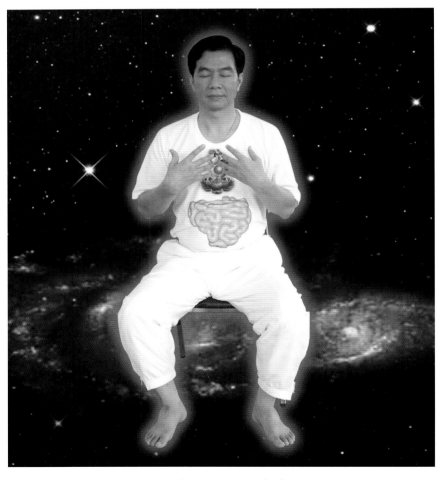

Fig. 7.25. Turn the senses in to the heart center.

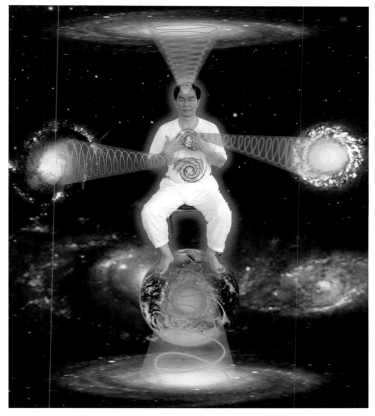

Fig. 7.26. Loving energy grows in the heart.

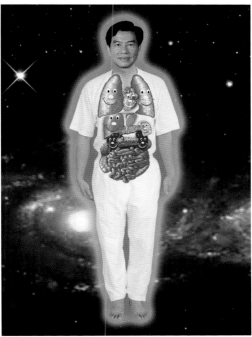

Fig. 7.27. When the heart is relieved of its daily load and stress, all the organs smile!

Feel any hatred, arrogance, or impatience transform into loving energy as sincerity, honor, and respect grow in your heart. Try to maintain the feeling of the heart's sound as long as you can after practice.

Repeat the steps from 3 to 6 times. Practice more to relieve sore throats, cold sores, swollen gums or tongue, jumpiness, moodiness, and heart disease.

 ## The Spleen's Sound: Fifth Cosmic Healing Sound

The spleen's sound is the earth sound, activating the energy of the stomach, the pancreas, and the spleen.

Characteristics

Associated organs: Pancreas, stomach
Element: Earth
Season: Indian summer
Color: Yellow
Emotion: Worry
Virtues: Fairness, openness
Parts of the body: Lips, mouth

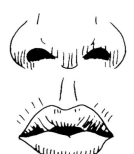

Fig. 7.28. Exhale on the sound "who-o-o-o-o-o."

Senses: Taste

Taste: Sweet, neutral

Sound: Who-o-o-o-o-o (from the throat, guttural) (fig. 7.28)

◈ Position and Practice

1. Sit comfortably with your back straight, your hands resting on your spleen, and your eyes closed. Smile down to your stomach and spleen until you feel you are in touch with them. Be aware of the quality of the energy in the stomach and the spleen. Picture a yellow light, the golden satiated light of Indian summer, a stable light (fig. 7.29).

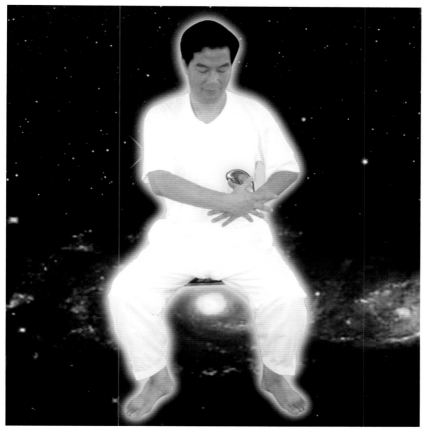

Fig. 7.29. Smile to the spleen.

2. Take a deep breath, open the eyes, move the arms to the front, and place the three middle fingers of both hands just beneath the sternum on the left side of the rib cage (fig. 7.30).

    Look up and gently press your fingers under the rib cage, pushing your stomach or spleen to the back and your middle back outward as you exhale, first saying out loud, and eventually subvocally, the sound "who-o-o-o-o-o." This is more guttural, or "throaty" than the kidneys' sound. Unlike blowing out a candle, this sound originates from within the chest, rather than from the mouth.

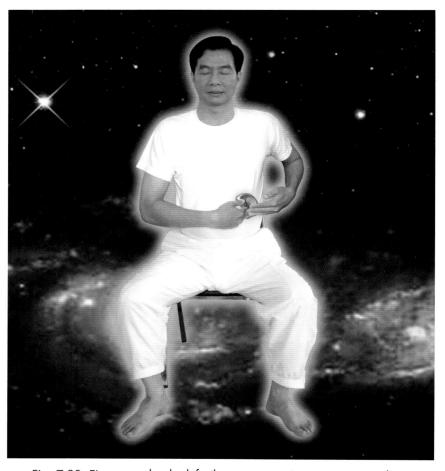

Fig. 7.30. Fingers under the left rib cage preparing to press on spleen, pancreas, and stomach

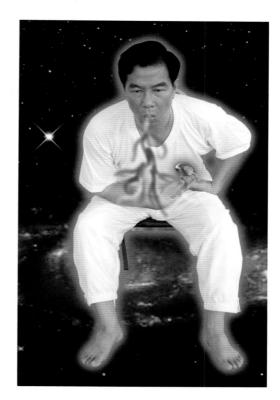

Fig. 7.31. Feel the
spleen's sound vibrate.

Feel the spleen's sound vibrate the vocal cords (fig. 7.31). Feel the sound start to move the energy in the stomach and the spleen, and feel that all excess heat and toxins are expelled from the stomach and the spleen as the sac around them is compressed.

3. After you have fully exhaled, move the arms outward, embracing the earth, and scoop up the yellow light. Pour this light into the stomach and spleen. Bring the arms and the hands to the stomach or the spleen. Radiate the yellow light, fairness, openness, and stability into the stomach and the spleen (see fig. 7.32 on page 144).

4. Rest, close your eyes, and be aware of your stomach and spleen. Smile to them and imagine that you are still making the spleen's sound. Feel the vibration of the sound moving and cleaning the energy in the stomach and the spleen.

Breathe normally, and see your stomach and spleen glow

with a yellow light. This will strengthen these organs and activate openness, fairness, and stability in your stomach and spleen. With each breath, try to feel that the warm yellow light is replacing the excess hot, toxic energy and any worries in these organs.

5. Nurture good emotions. This is the most important part of this practice. Take as much time as you need to get in touch with the stomach and the spleen. When you get rid of the excess heat and

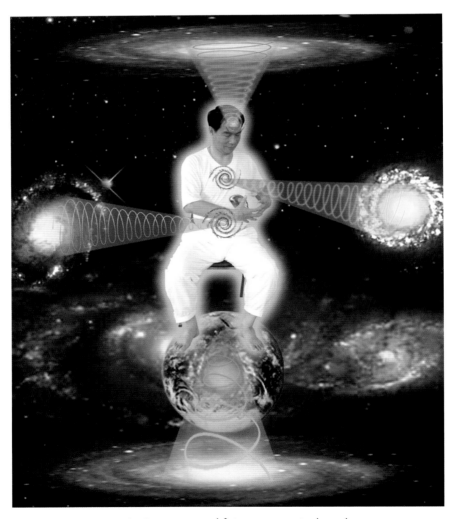

Fig. 7.32. Openness and fairness grow in the spleen.

let the yellow earth energy expand in the stomach and the spleen, good emotional qualities will have room to grow. Feel the fairness, openness, balance, and harmony grow in these organs, transforming any worry in them. Try to maintain the feeling of the spleen's sound as long as you can after practice.

Repeat the steps from 3 to 6 times. Practice more to eliminate indigestion, nausea, and diarrhea.

The Triple Warmer's Sound: Sixth Cosmic Healing Sound

The triple warmer refers to the three energy centers of the body: the upper section (brain, heart, and lungs) is hot; the middle section (liver, kidneys, stomach, pancreas, and spleen) is warm; and the lower section (large and small intestines, bladder, and sexual organs) is cool.

The sound "hee-e-e-e-e-e" (fig. 7.33) serves to balance the temperature of the three levels by bringing hot energy down to the lower center and cold energy up to the higher center. Specifically, hot energy from the area of the heart is moved to the colder sexual region, and cold energy from the lower abdomen is moved up to the heart's region.

Fig. 7.33. Make the "hee-e-e-e-e-e" sound on exhalation.

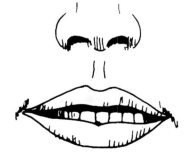

⟲ Position and Practice

1. Lie on your back or lean back in the chair (fig. 7.34). Smile, move your arms up to gather the chi (fig. 7.35), and bring your arms and hands to your face. As you make the "hee-e-e-e-e-e" sound on exhalation, let the arms slowly move down the body bringing the energy down from the crown to the feet (fig. 7.36).

2. Inhale fully into all three cavities: chest, solar plexus, and lower abdomen, and then exhale completely. Exhale with the sound "hee-e-e-e-e-e" subvocally, first flattening your chest, then your solar plexus, and finally your lower abdomen. Imagine a large roller pressing out your breath, and move the hot energy down as the

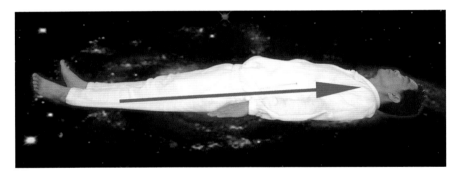

Fig. 7.34. Rest by breathing normally and focus on the triple warmer's sound.

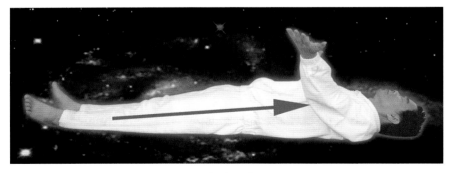

Fig. 7.35. Gather the energy.

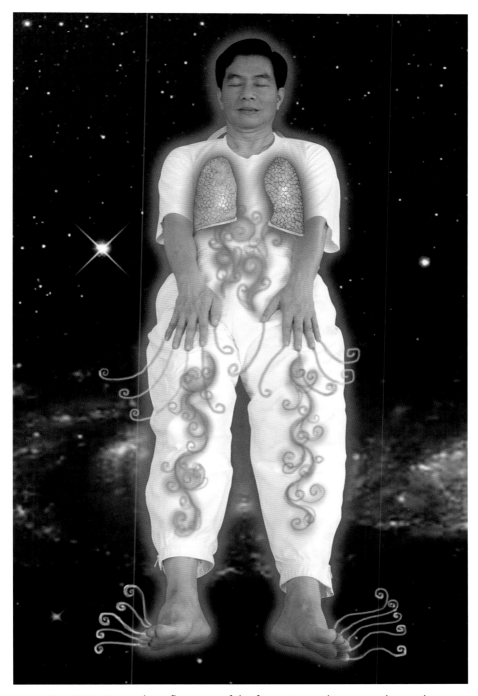

Fig. 7.36. Excess heat flows out of the fingertips and toes into the earth.

arms move from your head down to your lower tan tien (figs. 7.37 to 7.39).

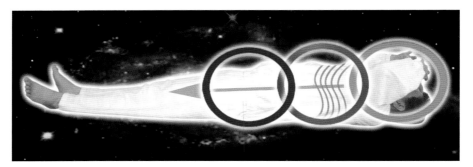

Fig. 7.37. Upper level

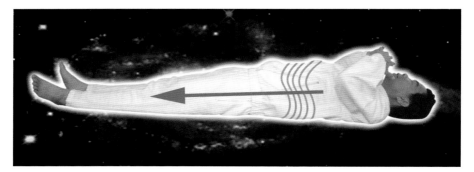

Fig. 7.38. Middle level

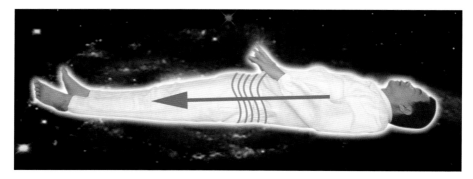

Fig. 7.39. Lower level

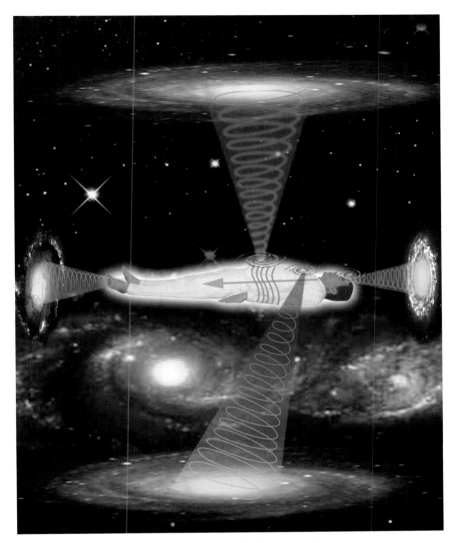

Fig. 7.40. Rest and absorb the cosmic forces.

3. Rest and concentrate (fig. 7.40). When you have fully exhaled, focus on the entire digestive tract.

Repeat the steps from 3 to 6 times. Practice more to relieve insomnia and stress. Note that the triple warmer's sound can be done lying down to facilitate falling asleep.

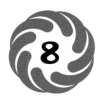

Taoist Emotional Recycling
The Practice

CHOOSE YOUR TOPIC

If this is your first time trying this practice you may want to just go through the process with no particular topic in mind. You can, in fact, use this technique over and over without ever focusing deliberately on any particular issue. You can just wait to see what comes up as you go through it and thereby work both in a preventive and a treatment mode. You can use the process to prevent the pileup that leads to depression, anxiety, and addiction.

Otherwise, take some time to figure out which topic you want to address first. Keep in mind that even if you choose what seems like a harmless or minor topic to address, you cannot know ahead of time how many more emotionally charged issues are attached to that one and will come up in the process. If you are having trouble choosing between a few topics, be aware that there is a chance that some or all of those topics may be connected and therefore it is not so critical which issue you address first. It is also important to realize that all of the issues can be addressed eventually and so the first topic does not have to be somehow more important than the others.

If you are still having trouble focusing on your topic you might want to read the set of questions in the section titled "Open Questions" in the next chapter.

CHOOSE WHERE YOU WANT TO START

To access the issue and its energetic counterpart in your system, you will need to pick an aspect of the issue that stands out in your mind; you will focus on this as your starting point. It can be a picture that stands out or, if visualizing does not come easily for you, it can be a feeling that you had at the time, a thought you have had about yourself since the issue arose, or some sound or smell that you remember. "Where the mind goes, the chi follows," so whatever you choose to focus on will bring energy to that aspect, which is the beginning of the process of transforming that experience into something that feels better.

Make sure that whatever you choose to focus on is something that you actually experienced, not something that you remember about the incident but did not actually experience at the time. For example, if you can see yourself in the picture you choose, it is not the right picture. Unless you were looking in a mirror at the time, you did not see yourself. Also, do not skip steps or try to speed up the process. You may end up spending a lot of time on particular areas of your body. If the issue is primarily stored in one or a few areas, it does not make sense to rush through that part. Give that part of your body the attention it deserves so it can heal.

PREPARATION

In order to be ready to digest unresolved experiences that are stored in your system, you should be committed, relaxed, and detoxified. Learning and practicing the Tao basics given in the previous chapter—Inner Smile, Microcosmic Orbit, and Six Healing Sounds—will ensure that the major energetic pathways are open and your chi level is strong enough to receive the benefits of this practice. It might also be advisable to hold a grounding stone (such as black obsidian) in your receiving hand (the opposite to your writing hand) to help you stay calm in the process and keep your energy level up enough to see the process to completion.

Commit to the Process

The type of commitment that is most effective for this process is unwavering commitment without reservation. Wishing or hoping that things will get better or telling yourself that you have to do it is not as effective as deciding that you will do whatever it will take to make sure that the troubling issues in your life are resolved. Your mind and body are connected. When you make that kind of commitment, you are already preparing your stuck energy to be broken apart.

Right Attitude

Make a conscious commitment to be ready to let go of the issue, even if the emotions that come up along the way are upsetting. Convince yourself that you do not need to hold on to the negative feelings that are associated with that issue in order to be the unique person that you are. Be aware that you may experience negative emotions soon after you begin the processing. That is actually a good sign. The emotions often need to come up before they can be released. Letting go is not just an emotional process. It can also be accomplished physically through tears, yawning, belching, flatulence, and any other process that expels waste out of the body.

However, also commit to the idea that you will take a break or stop and search out professional guidance if you become overwhelmed in the process. The process can be uncomfortable, but it is supposed to be about healing, not ripping and tearing. The purpose of this technique is to help you rid yourself of upsetting feelings, not give you more of them. If you are skeptical that this process can help you, just put that skepticism aside for the duration of the exercise so you can create the best possible climate for the process to work. Be ready to be taken on a journey that will not always, or maybe not often, make sense. Be prepared to follow the process no matter where it takes you.

Detoxify

Stress and fear come from your kidneys when they are out of balance. Gently rub your kidneys in the back for about thirty seconds (fig. 8.1). For more stimulation, try rubbing with your hands in loose fists. Drink some water to clean out your kidneys and help them relax. If you have access to a professional who provides colonics, that would also be very helpful. Remove stimulants such as cigarettes, caffeine, and illicit drugs from your lifestyle as much as possible so your system can be as calm as possible before you start the process. Then you will have less risk of becoming overwhelmed during the treatment.

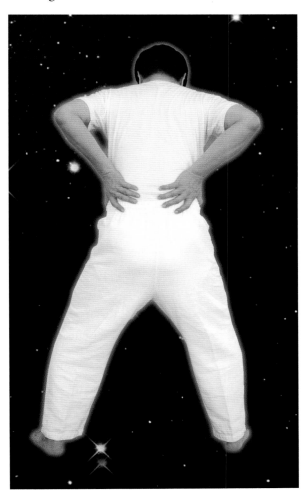

Fig. 8.1. Rub your kidneys to promote detoxification.

Lights, Smells, and Sound

Keep soft lighting in the room during the exercise or turn the lights off completely. If you like, use some aromatherapy to help you to remain relaxed through the process. Scents like lemongrass and peppermint are soothing. Incense is suitable in a ventilated area, but the smoke from it might be distracting if you are in a small, confined space. Refrain from using sounds to help you relax unless they are soft nature sounds. Music might be relaxing at other times, but during this exercise it might make it more difficult to focus your mind on the memories that you are trying to address.

If you have training in the Taoist Cosmic Healing practice and Chi Nei Tsang you could prepare the room as you would for those practices to ensure that the healing forces are present and that you are in a protected circle.

Slow Down and Relax

Give yourself enough time to wind down and loosen up your body before you move to the next steps. The calmer you are before you start processing away past experiences, the more room you will have inside yourself to process. If you are "halfway to a boil" before you start, it will take very little to push you beyond your limits. Making sure your body is loose before you start will increase the likelihood that you will be able to release the toxins that are trapped inside you and connected to the issue you are addressing. If your body is tight, you are still holding tight to the issue, and it will be more difficult for it to leave your system.

To get into the right state for the work, first pick a quiet place to sit, in which you feel comfortable and will not be interrupted. Make sure that you do not have social obligations to meet right after this exercise. You may feel tired and will probably feel more able to sink into the exercise if you know that you will have the option to relax and be alone after you are finished. Breathe in your lower abdomen. Use slow, soft, and gentle but full breaths. Inhale and exhale through your nose. There is no need to strain. Just allow your abdomen to fill and empty fully, like a newborn baby fresh into the world. As you breathe you are flushing out your system and giving it a message that everything is fine.

❷ *Beginning Seated Position*

1. Sit on the edge of a chair with your feet flat on the floor. That way you will not lose energy out of your feet; you can draw energy from the earth, and less of your body will be cut off from the earth's energy.
2. Clasp your hands gently in your lap. Then you will not lose energy out of your hands (fig. 8.2a).
3. Put the tip of your tongue lightly on the roof of your mouth in the indentation of your palate behind your gum-line (fig. 8.2b) and keep your mouth closed. That energetically joins the two halves of

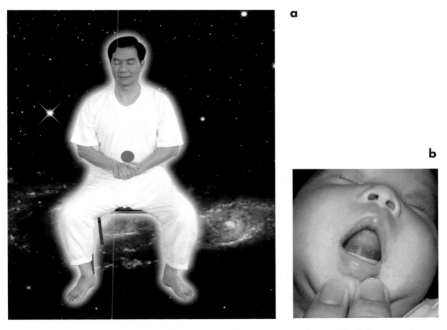

Fig. 8.2. Beginning seated position with tongue on the roof of the mouth

your jaw and the two vessels in the Microcosmic Orbit. Now your body is one big circuit that is connected to the earth and its energy.

☯ *Warm Up Your Lower Tan Tien and Kidneys*

To protect, prepare, and heal your kidneys and stop the downward spiral in your energy, you need to make sure that your kidneys and intestines are warm and soft.

1. Put your hands on your lower abdomen, one palm on top of the other.
2. Spiral your palms in a clockwise direction for men and counterclockwise for women, making small circles that get progressively larger. Continue until your abdomen and kidneys feel nice and warm and soft.
3. Spiral the energy in your lower tan tien to warm it and prepare for the work to come.

If you want to be more thorough and systematic in your relaxation process, you can try the following exercise.

☯ *Three Minds into One Mind*

1. Pick a comfortable and quiet place to sit. Put your feet flat on the floor. Breathe gently but fully in your lower abdomen. Smile so that you look like the Mona Lisa. Lift up the corners of your mouth and eyes.
2. Lightly touch your fingertips to the middle of your forehead (not in between your eyebrows). Smile, breathe, and focus where your fingers are. Allow the feeling to grow, expand, or focus. Your fingers are touching the first mind, your Center of Happiness.
3. Then slowly draw your fingers down the middle of your face and follow your fingers with your mind. This brings some of the energy

from your first mind with your fingers. Move them over your nose, lips, and chin.

4. Move them down your neck and then over to the left and down to your heart. Keep your fingertips there for a moment while you smile and breathe and focus on your heart. This mixes the energy from the first mind with the energy in the second mind, the sac around your heart, your Center of Peace (fig. 8.3). Feel your heart warm and go soft. We call this "melting the ice."

5. Now move your fingers from your heart toward the midline of your body. Then start moving your fingers slowly down your body and again follow your fingers with your mind. Keep smiling and breathing as you go. Stop when your fingers are about 1½ inches below your navel. That is your third mind, the Center of Control. You are now mixing the energy from the first two minds with the third mind.

6. Put your hands, one palm on top of the other, on top of your third mind. Smile, breathe, and think about where your hands are. Allow the feeling to expand. Notice that your hands become warm quickly.

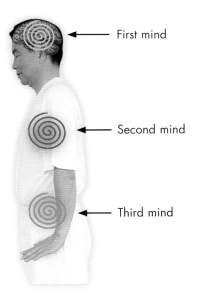

First mind

Second mind

Third mind

Fig. 8.3. Three minds

PUTTING HEALTHY LIMITS ON
YOUR TREATMENT

Typically an hour or an hour and a half is the maximum amount of processing that is recommended for a person to do in a single session. Be aware that you can stop whenever you want when you practice on your own, so your treatment session could be as short as ten minutes in duration if that is all the time or energy you have. Just make sure you do the appropriate healing sound a few times at the end of the session so you can leave the exercise feeling as calm as possible. If you use eye movements in the treatment and your eyes become sore or tired from the movements, close your eyelids and gently rub on and around your eyeballs between treatment sets. Be careful not to wear yourself out too much. Your intention to release yourself from the issue might be good but it is important to honor your limits. Otherwise you may wear yourself out to the point where you will not feel like continuing for a long time, maybe longer than if you had just approached the topic at a manageable pace.

Make sure you do not have any more negative feelings come up when you think about the picture you started with before you move on to the next part of the body. If you can feel energy moving after the processing but the feeling is not negative then that is fine. You can move on to the next activity.

If you cannot completely resolve the negative feelings after repeated attempts, you may need to search your mind for an earlier or separate but related event to process after you have done as much as you can to address the one you are focusing on now. Sometimes related events are stored in different places or in different ways, so you need to address them separately.

THINGS TO CONSIDER BEFORE YOU
BEGIN PROCESSING YOUR ISSUE

Not everyone is comfortable with the eye movements. If you can use them but you find that your eyes get sore when you first start practicing or periodically during the treatment, remember that you can stop at times, close your eyelids, and lightly rub on your eyeballs to loosen the muscles that help you to do the eye movements. If you cannot use the eye movements due to vertigo or some other condition, you can put your hands, palm on top of palm, on each body part and move them in the directions that you would have moved your eyes. You do not have to press your hands hard against your body but do make clear contact with it. People who have training in Taoist Cosmic Healing may try spiraling without touching their bodies. If you can do it, move your eyes and palms together. That way you will be able to focus in on the material you are trying to neutralize from two sensory angles.

Remember that everyone has unique reactions to this practice. You may notice nothing in particular as you do the processing. That does not mean it will not work. However, do not be surprised if other material comes up while you are doing the processing. This material may be clearly related to the starting point or it may seem unrelated. Everything that comes up is being processed as well, so be glad that it arises.

Some people who started with an image to focus on will notice that it becomes blurry or faded over time. That is a good sign.

Also, do not be concerned if you cannot hold on to your starting image or focus on your body part and starting point throughout the processing. The focus at the beginning is important to set the stage for the healing to occur, but once you start the hand or eye movements the process happens naturally. Let it flow.

The eye and hand movements may seem difficult at first. Aside from the fact that this process is new to you, they are also difficult because the issue is still dark, thick, and heavy. As you work through your chosen issue it will feel clearer, lighter, and softer and your hand and eye movements will become easier as a result.

Finally, do not focus too much on the number of sets or repetitions of each part of the process. If you focus too much on counting, it will take away from your ability to focus on the issue and may limit how much benefit you will receive from the exercise. The exact number of movements that you use is not critical to the success or failure of this approach. Think, for example, about trying to move your hand in water in a sink. How many times would you need to swish the water back and forth before it moves on its own? There is no exact or magic number for that. The same kind of thinking applies when you spiral your eyes and hands. So especially when you first start practicing, try not to be too focused on the technical details of the process. Just let it unfold.

Processing in Your Center of Happiness

As you do this Taoist Emotional Recycling practice your eyes will move back and forth and in spirals in sync with the spiraling of your hands. As you move your eyes and spiral your hands it will be important to allow your mind and body to do whatever they want without trying to steer your reactions toward something that makes sense to you. It does not even matter if the reactions or memories that you experience as a result of the processing are accurate. Trust your body and mind to know how best to handle the situation.

Pay attention to what you are thinking, feeling, picturing, or sensing in your body as the processing continues. If you are not noticing anything or you get dizzy, you are probably spiraling too quickly.

Take breaks in between each batch of eye movements until you feel calm enough to continue, but do not let your mind wander too far away from what you were experiencing during the eye movements that you just completed.

Opening Yourself to the Issue

1. Breathe in your lower abdomen. Smile. Lift the corners of your eyes and mouth like the Mona Lisa.
2. Think about the aspect of the issue that you chose to focus on to start. Bring it as vividly to your memory as you can. Use your inner senses to see, hear, smell, touch, and taste it.

3. Smile to your heart. Feel energy moving on top of your head. That is letting you know that the nine energetic mountains on top of your head are open and connecting to the violet light.

✪ Processing the Issue

1. Close your eyes, focus on the middle of your forehead, and mentally place the chosen aspect of your issue in the middle of your forehead. If you are using your hands, put one palm on top of the other with the inside of your palms facing your forehead.
2. Move your eyes and/or your palms left and right, looking left and right up inside your brain. Do that for about 18 sets. Moving your eyes left and right, one time each, constitutes one set.
3. With your eyelids still closed, slowly spiral your eyes and/or palms, while continuing to focus on the issue in the middle of your forehead, so that you make small circles that become progressively larger in a counterclockwise direction (fig. 8.4). Counterclockwise means

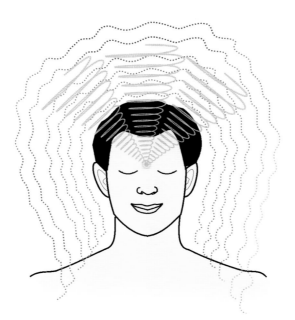

Fig. 8.4. Process the issue in your Center of Happiness.

you move up on the left side and down on the right. Ideally you will make 36 revolutions, but any multiple of nine will work. Make sure your eyes and/or your hands are moving very slowly. It should take a couple of seconds for each revolution of the spiral.

4. Then reverse the direction of the spiraling and make circles that get progressively smaller for a maximum of 24 revolutions. Any multiple of six revolutions will work.

5. Rest for a minute. Take your mind off the issue. Then repeat the left-and-right and spiraling movements. You can focus on the same starting point at the beginning of each set or start the next set with the last thought, picture, feeling, or body sensation that occurred at the end of the previous set.

6. Rest. Continue the repetitions until you no longer feel any negative reaction in the middle of your forehead when you focus on your beginning image, feeling, or sound. After you complete a set of eye and/or hand movements and you think the issue might be neutralized in the forehead, close your eyes and focus on the starting point you have been using. If there are no mind or body reactions to the starting point then you can probably move on to the next body area to be processed.

7. However, before you move on, check to see if you still have any negative beliefs about yourself—like "I am bad," "I am unworthy," or "I cannot stand up for myself"—when you think about the issue. If you do, focus on that belief and the starting point that you used for the exercise and do more sets of back-and-forth movements and then spirals in the same manner as before until the belief does not feel true to you at all.

Once the negative feelings are gone, you will probably notice that good feelings start to fill you up automatically. Taking this step helps to make sure that your faith in yourself is no longer being hampered at all by this issue.

If you become too emotional or feel too much heat in your brain during the processing you should stop and make the lungs' sound (sss-s-s-s-s-s) quietly. Take a slow, deep breath and make the sound while you exhale completely. Then wait. Then do it again. Do it a few times until you feel cool and calm. You should also make the sound again before you move on to the next part of the treatment.

Activate and Transform Your Center of Peace

Even if you do not feel any upset feelings, tension, or pain in your body after transforming the energy in your Center of Happiness, you should still complete the exercise. As you work with the individual internal organs you will likely notice that more negative emotions connected to the issue you have chosen have been stored within your organs, but you will not feel these emotions until you focus on them in the right way.

1. Focus on the same starting point that you used when you cleared the emotion out of your Center of Happiness.
2. Smile and focus on your heart. See it inside your body. See the color red around your heart. At first the red color may be dark, cloudy, or murky. As you continue to smile and focus on your heart, it will become a clearer and brighter red color. The darkness in the red color is toxic energy. As you smile to it you transform that toxic energy into healthy, virtuous energy. You are transforming hastiness, impatience, hatred, and cruelty into joy, happiness, and love.
3. Keep smiling to your heart until the red color will not get any clearer and brighter (see fig. 8.5 on page 164).
4. Put one palm on top of the other and place your hands palms down on your heart. Think about the aspect of the issue that you have chosen and mentally place it inside, or on top of, your heart.
5. Now, while focusing on the issue in your heart, close your eyes and slowly move them and/or your hands back and forth from left to right for about 18 sets.
6. With your eyelids still closed and continuing to focus on the issue

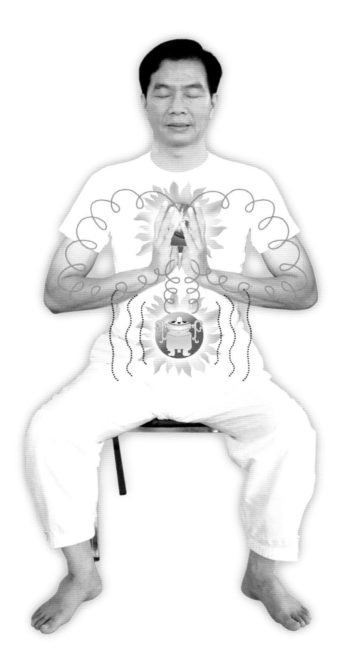

Fig. 8.5. Activate and transform your Center of Peace.

in your heart, slowly spiral your eyes and/or your hands so that you make small circles that become progressively larger in a counter-clockwise direction. Counterclockwise means you move up on the left side and down on the right. Ideally you will make 36 revolutions, but any multiple of nine will work. Make sure your eyes and/or your hands are moving very slowly. It should take a couple of seconds for each revolution of the spiral.

7. Then reverse the direction of the spiraling and make circles that get progressively smaller for a maximum of 24 revolutions. Any multiple of six revolutions will work.

8. Rest for a minute. Take your mind off the issue. Then repeat the left-and-right and spiraling movements. You can focus on the same starting point at the beginning of each set or start the next set with the last thought, picture, feeling, or body sensation that occurred at the end of the previous set.

9. Rest. Continue the repetitions until you no longer feel any negative reaction in your mind or in your heart when you focus on your beginning image, feeling, or sound. After you complete a set of eye and/or hand movements and you think the issue might be neutralized in your heart, close your eyes and focus on the starting point you have been using. If there are no mind or body reactions to the starting point then you can move on to the next body area to be processed.

10. Check to see if you still have any negative beliefs about yourself—like "I am bad," "I am unworthy," or "I cannot stand up for myself"—when you think about the issue. If you do, focus on that belief and the starting point that you used for the exercise and do more sets of back-and-forth movements and then spirals in the same manner as before until the belief does not feel true to you at all.

Once the negative feelings are gone, you will probably notice that good feelings start to fill you up automatically.

Whenever you feel yourself getting upset during the processing, you can use the healing sound for the heart (haw-w-w-w-w) to cool your heart and keep yourself calm. Make sure you do the sound at least a couple of times at the completion of the spiraling for this section.

❂ Dissolve the Connection between Your Center of Peace and Your Center of Happiness

In addition to neutralizing the emotional energy for your chosen issue in your heart area, we also want to make sure that any residual connection between the issue and your heart is removed. Think about a computer again. What we want to do now is akin to dissolving the connection between your hardware (the mind, which controls access to programs) and your software (the organs, which process and transform material into new forms). In this case, the software is your heart.

Return to the forehead and complete the exercise while focusing on your Center of Happiness again. This removes the link between the brain and the heart. This process usually takes only one set of hand and/or eye movements.

❂ Neutralize the Issue in Your Spleen

1. Now move your hands to your left side under your ribs. That is where your spleen is. Put one palm on top of the other and then place your hands palms down on your spleen. Smile and focus on your spleen. Look inside and see it.

2. See a yellow color around your spleen. As you smile to your spleen, you are transforming toxic energy into virtuous energy. You are transforming negative thinking, overthinking, and worry into openness and trust. Smiling to your spleen will allow any dark and cloudy color in the spleen to become clearer and brighter.

3. Keep smiling to your spleen until the yellow color does not become any cleaner (fig. 8.6). Then mentally place the aspect of your issue that you have chosen into, or on top of, your spleen.

4. Now close your eyes and move them and/or your hands left and

progressively smaller for a maximum of 24 revolutions. Any multiple of six revolutions will work.

7. Rest for a minute. Take your mind off the issue. Then repeat the left-and-right and spiraling eye and/or hand movements. You can focus on the same starting point at the beginning of each set or start the next set with the last thought, picture, feeling, or body sensation that occurred at the end of the previous set.

8. Rest. Continue the repetitions until you no longer feel any negative reaction in your mind or in your spleen when you focus on your beginning image, feeling, or sound. After you complete a set of eye and/or hand movements and you think the issue might be neutralized in your spleen, close your eyes and focus on the starting point you have been using. If there are no mind or body reactions to the starting point then you can probably move on to the next body area to be processed.

9. However, before you move on, check to see if you still have any negative beliefs about yourself—like "I am bad," "I am unworthy," or "I cannot stand up for myself"—when you think about the issue. If you do, focus on that belief and the starting point that you used for the exercise and do more sets of back-and-forth movements and then spirals in the same manner as before until the belief does not feel true to you at all.

Once the negative feelings are gone, you will probably notice that good feelings start to fill you up automatically.

Use the healing sound for the spleen (who-o-o-o-o-o) to calm yourself down and cool off your spleen as you work on it. Make sure you do the sound at least a couple of times at the completion of the spiraling for this section before you move on to the next one.

❧ Dissolve the Connection Between Your Center of Happiness and Your Spleen

Now go back to your forehead and use both the back-and-forth movements and the spiraling movements to clear any reactions that have come up since you worked on your spleen. That will remove the link between your spleen and your brain for this issue.

 ## Transform the Issue in Your Lungs

1. Put one palm on each of your lungs. Smile to your lungs. Look inside and see your lungs. See white around your lungs. Do not be alarmed if the white color looks dark, cloudy, or murky. The darkness is just toxic energy that you can transform into virtuous energy. As you smile to your lungs you will be able to transform those toxins and change the toxic emotions of grief, sadness, loss, and depression into the virtues of courage and righteousness (fig. 8.7).

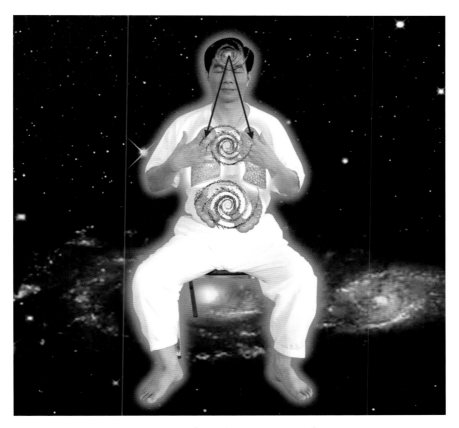

Fig. 8.7. Transform the issue in your lungs.

2. Once you have transformed as much of that energy as possible with the power of your focused smiling energy, focus on the aspect of the issue that you have chosen and mentally place it inside, or on top of, one of your lungs.

3. Close your eyes and move your eyes and/or your hands slowly left and right for about 18 sets.

4. With your eyelids still closed and continuing to focus on the issue in your lungs, slowly spiral your eyes and/or your hands so that you make small circles that become progressively larger in a counterclockwise direction, moving up on the left side and down on the right. Ideally you will make 36 revolutions, but any multiple of nine will work. Make sure your eyes and/or your hands are moving very slowly. It should take a couple of seconds for each revolution of the spiral.

5. Then reverse the direction of the spiraling and make circles that get progressively smaller for a maximum of 24 revolutions. Any multiple of six revolutions will work.

6. Rest for a minute. Take your mind off the issue. Then repeat the left-and-right and spiraling movements. You can focus on the same starting point at the beginning of each set or start the next set with the last thought, picture, feeling, or body sensation that occurred at the end of the previous set.

7. Rest. Continue the repetitions until you no longer feel any negative reaction in your mind or in the lung where you placed the issue when you focus on your beginning image, feeling, or sound. After you complete a set of eye and/or hand movements and you think the issue might be neutralized in your lungs, close your eyes and focus on the starting point you have been using. If there are no mind or body reactions to the starting point then you can probably move on to the next body area to be processed.

8. However, before you move on, check to see if you still have any negative beliefs about yourself—like "I am bad," "I am unworthy," or "I cannot stand up for myself"—when you think about the issue. If you do, focus on that belief and the starting point that you used

for the exercise and do more sets of back-and-forth movements and then spirals in the same manner as before until the belief does not feel true to you at all.

Once the negative feelings are gone, you will probably notice that good feelings start to fill you up automatically.

To keep your lungs cool and to keep yourself calm, you can use the healing sound for your lungs (sss-s-s-s-s) during the processing in between sets of spiraling. Make sure you do the sound at least a couple of times at the end of this section before you move on to the next one.

Dissolve the Connection between Your Center of Happiness and Your Lungs

Now return once again to your forehead and process the issue out of that area as you have before. That will remove the link between your brain and your lungs regarding this issue.

Process Negative Emotions Out of Your Kidneys

1. Smile and focus on your kidneys. Put one palm on each kidney to make a connection with them. See them inside your body. See a blue color around your kidneys. The blue color may not be completely clear and bright at first, but as you smile to your kidneys it will improve.
2. When it has improved all that it can with the power of your inner smile, focus on the aspect of your issue that you have chosen and mentally place it in or on either of your kidneys (see fig. 8.8 on page 172).
3. Close your eyes and move your eyes and/or your hands left and right for about 18 sets while you look inside your kidney at the part of the issue that you chose.
4. With your eyelids still closed and continuing to focus on the issue

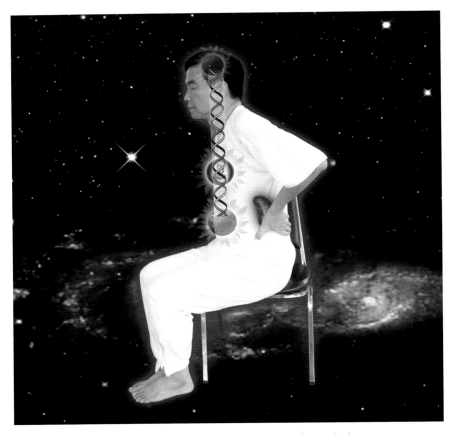

Fig. 8.8. Process negative emotions out of your kidneys.

in your kidney, slowly spiral your eyes and/or your hands so that you make small circles that become progressively larger in a counterclockwise direction, moving up on the left side and down on the right. Ideally you will make 36 revolutions, but any multiple of nine will work. Make sure your eyes and/or your hands are moving very slowly. It should take a couple of seconds for each revolution of the spiral.

5. Then reverse the direction of the spiraling and make circles that get progressively smaller for a maximum of 24 revolutions. Any multiple of six revolutions will work.

6. Rest for a minute. Take your mind off the issue. Then repeat the

left-and-right and spiraling. You can focus on the same starting point at the beginning of each set or start the next set with the last thought, picture, feeling, or body sensation that occurred at the end of the previous set.

7. Rest. Continue the repetitions until you no longer feel any negative reaction in your mind or in the kidney where you placed the issue when you focus on your beginning image, feeling, or sound. After you complete a set of eye and/or hand movements and you think the issue might be neutralized in the kidneys, close your eyes and focus on the starting point you have been using. If there are no mind or body reactions to the starting point then you can probably move on to the next body area to be processed.

8. However, before you move on, check to see if you still have any negative beliefs about yourself—like "I am bad," "I am unworthy," or "I cannot stand up for myself"—when you think about the issue. If you do, focus on that belief and the starting point that you used for the exercise and do more sets of back-and-forth movements and then spirals in the same manner as before until the belief does not feel true to you at all.

Once the negative feelings are gone, you will probably notice that good feelings start to fill you up automatically.

You can keep yourself calm and your kidneys cool during the processing in this section by using the kidneys' healing sound (choo-oo-oo-oo). At the very least, do the sound a couple of times at the end of this section.

Dissolve the Connection Between Your Kidneys and Your Center of Happiness

Now return to your forehead and process the issue out of that area in the same manner you have done before. That removes the link between your brain and your kidneys regarding this issue.

Rebalancing and Purifying the Energy in Your Sexual Organs

1. Put one palm on top of the other and place your hands palms down on your sexual organs. Smile to your sexual organs. See them with a pink color around them. As you smile to them the pink color will become clearer and brighter as toxins are transformed into the virtues that come from your sexual organs. This can help transform some trauma and restore your overall vitality.

2. Once the pink color has become as clear and bright as possible from smiling to your sexual organs, you can mentally place the chosen aspect of your issue into them (fig. 8.9). Picture it or feel it inside, or on top of, your sexual organs. Do not be concerned if the issue that you are working on is not of a sexual nature. We are working in this area because we want to neutralize any emotional content coming from the sexual organs that has been affected by this issue.

3. Now close your eyes and move your eyes and/or your hands back

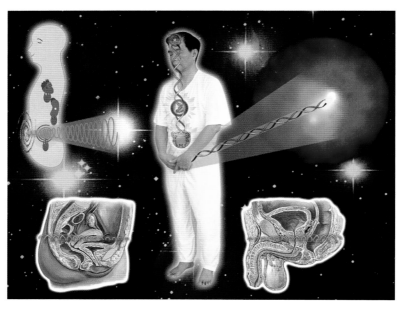

Fig. 8.9. Rebalancing and purifying the energy in your sexual organs

and forth for about 18 sets. Notice what happens inside you.

4. With your eyelids still closed and continuing to focus on the issue in your sexual organs, slowly spiral your eyes and/or your hands so that you make small circles that become progressively larger in a counterclockwise direction, moving up on the left side and down on the right. Ideally you will make 36 revolutions, but any multiple of nine will work. Make sure your eyes and/or your hands are moving very slowly. It should take a couple of seconds for each revolution of the spiral.

5. Then reverse the direction of the spiraling and make circles that get progressively smaller for a maximum of 24 revolutions. Any multiple of six revolutions will work.

6. Rest for a minute. Take your mind off the issue. Then repeat the left-and-right and spiraling movements. You can focus on the same starting point at the beginning of each set or start the next set with the last thought, picture, feeling, or body sensation that occurred at the end of the previous set.

7. Rest. Continue the repetitions until you no longer feel any negative reaction in your mind or in your sexual organs when you focus on your beginning image, feeling, or sound. After you complete a set of eye and/or hand movements and you think the issue might be neutralized in your sexual organs, close your eyes and focus on the starting point you have been using. If there are no mind or body reactions to the starting point then you can probably move on to the next body area to be processed.

8. However, before you move on, check to see if you still have any negative beliefs about yourself—like "I am bad," "I am unworthy," or "I cannot stand up for myself"—when you think about the issue. If you do, focus on that belief and the starting point that you used for the exercise and do more sets of back-and-forth movements and then spirals in the same manner as before until the belief does not feel true to you at all.

Once the negative feelings are gone, you will probably notice that good feelings start to fill you up automatically.

There is no designated healing sound for the sexual organs, but you can use the triple warmer's sound (hee-e-e-e-e-e), which works on the whole body, to keep yourself from becoming too hot or upset during the processing. If you do not need to use it during the processing, at least do it a couple of times at the end of this section so that you are as ready as possible to start the next one.

Dissolve the Connection between Your Sexual Organs and Your Center of Happiness

Now return to your forehead and process the issue in that area again in the same manner that you have done before in this exercise. That will remove the link between your sexual organs and your brain regarding this issue.

Digest and Recycle the Negative Energy in Your Liver

1. Your liver is a big triangular-shaped organ to the right side of your body under your ribs. Put one palm on top of the other and place your hands palms down on your liver. Smile to your liver. See it inside you. See a green color around it. As you smile to your liver you are transforming the toxic energy inside it. You are transforming anger, frustration, jealousy, and envy into generosity and kindness. Smile to your liver and watch the green color become brighter and clearer until it cannot improve any more that way (fig. 8.10).

2. Focus on the aspect of the issue that you have chosen and mentally place it inside, or on top of, your liver.

3. Now close your eyes and move your eyes and/or your hands back and forth for about 18 sets while you focus on the issue in your liver. Notice what happens.

4. With your eyelids still closed and continuing to focus on the issue in your liver, slowly spiral your eyes and/or your hands so that you

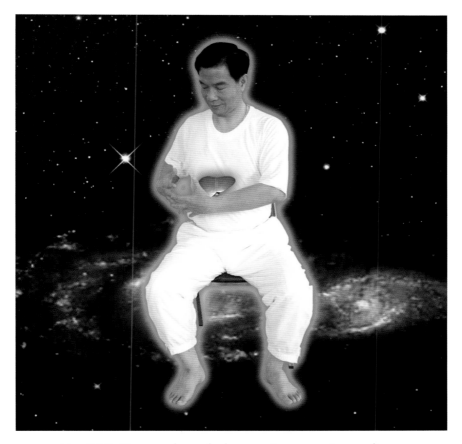

Fig. 8.10. Digest and recycle the negative energy in your liver.

make small circles that become progressively larger in a counter-clockwise direction, moving up on the left side and down on the right. Ideally you will make 36 revolutions, but any multiple of nine will work. Make sure your eyes and/or your hands are moving very slowly. It should take a couple of seconds for each revolution of the spiral.

5. Then reverse the direction of the spiraling and make circles that get progressively smaller for a maximum of 24 revolutions. Any multiple of six revolutions will work.

6. Rest for a minute. Take your mind off the issue. Then repeat the left-and-right and spiraling movements. You can focus on the same

starting point at the beginning of each set or start the next set with the last thought, picture, feeling, or body sensation that occurred at the end of the previous set.

7. Rest. Continue the repetitions until you no longer feel any negative reaction in your mind or in your liver when you focus on your beginning image, feeling, or sound. After you complete a set of eye and/or hand movements and you think the issue might be neutralized in your liver, close your eyes and focus on the starting point you have been using. If there are no mind or body reactions to the starting point then you can probably move on to the next body area to be processed.

8. However, before you move on, check to see if you still have any negative beliefs about yourself—like "I am bad," "I am unworthy," or "I cannot stand up for myself"—when you think about the issue. If you do, focus on that belief and the starting point that you used for the exercise and do more sets of back-and-forth movements and then spirals in the same manner as before until the belief does not feel true to you at all.

Once the negative feelings are gone, you will probably notice that good feelings start to fill you up automatically.

Do the healing sound for the liver (sh-h-h-h-h-h-h) a couple of times at the end of this section after you have finished with the spiraling. You can also use it during this section of the practice if you get too upset.

⊙ Dissolve the Connection Between Your Liver and Your Center of Happiness

Now return to your forehead and delete, recycle, and transform in that area again in the same manner that you have done previously. That will remove the link between your brain and your liver in connection to the issue you have been addressing.

Clean Up the Rest of Your Body

1. Now think about the issue that you are addressing and check over your entire body. Wherever you still feel something negative in your body, place your palms over that spot and process away the undigested energy in the same manner that you did for all of your organs.

2. After you have neutralized a spot that was still reacting to the issue, think about the issue again and re-check your body to see if a new area is reacting to it.

3. If you sense an area of discomfort, place your palms over that spot and process away the undigested energy in the same manner that you did for all of your organs.

4. Keep doing this until there are no other areas that feel tense, uncomfortable, or painful when you think about the issue. If you use your hands to do the processing you may need someone else to spiral for you if the discomfort moves to an area on your back that you cannot reach. Try putting your palms on your sacrum and the back of your head, even if you do not feel any particular discomfort there. Those areas tend to store emotions that are connected to events from your past.

Microcosmic Orbit

1. Use the Microcosmic Orbit meditation given in chapter 7 to circulate the transformed energy (see fig. 8.11 on page 180). Send the energy through the orbit to feed all the channels and share the healing you have done with your entire body.

2. To energize yourself, circulate the energy up the back and down the front; if you are tired, circulate it up the front and down the back.

3. To relax yourself, create a figure eight vertically between the top and bottom halves of your body to connect with eternity, and create a figure eight horizontally, going out from the center of your

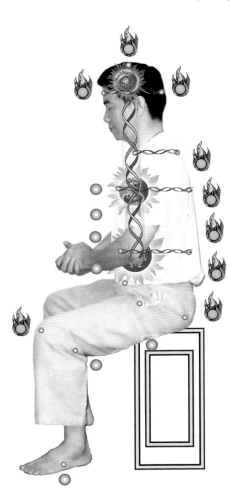

Fig. 8.11. You can use the Microcosmic Orbit to circulate the healthy energy you have created through your body and connect with the energy around you.

body to connect with infinity. Just focus your mind and move slowly through the pattern you chose.

Spiral to Transform and Store the Virtuous Energy in the Center of Control

1. Place your palms on top of your lower tan tien, about 1½ inches below your navel (fig. 8.12).
2. **Men:** Cover the navel with both palms, left over right. Massage with a spiraling motion clockwise 36 times (fig. 8.13).

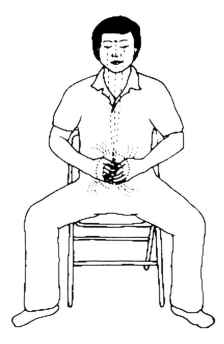

Fig. 8.12. Collecting and storing the energy

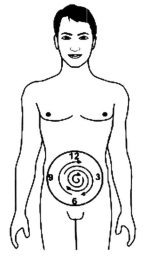

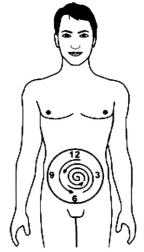

Men collect the energy by spiraling outward from the navel 36 times clockwise.

Then they spiral inward 24 times counterclockwise, ending at the navel.

Fig. 8.13. How men collect energy

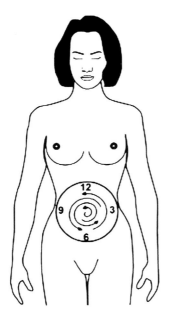
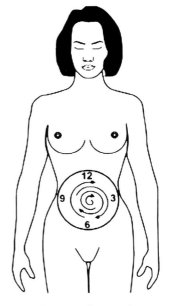

Women collect the energy by spiraling outward from the navel 36 times counterclockwise.

Then they spiral inward 24 times clockwise, ending at the navel.

Fig. 8.14. How women collect energy

Women: Cover the navel with both palms, right over left. Massage counterclockwise with a spiraling motion 36 times (fig. 8.14).

Men and women: Reverse directions, and spiral back into the navel 24 times. (Men spiral counterclockwise; women spiral clockwise.) Move closer to the navel with each cycle.

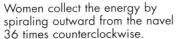 Rest and Recuperate

After you have finished the exercise, or finished as much as you can do for one day, take it easy for the rest of the day. You may feel quite drained at this point. You will be fine by the next day as long as you give yourself a chance for proper rest. You can keep using the Microcosmic Orbit to help rebalance your energy.

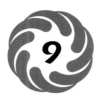

Helping Other People

If you complete the training to become certified in this practice, you can follow the same procedures to walk other people through the steps to heal themselves. Make sure you follow the procedures exactly. Do not skip steps. They are all important.

The Universal Healing Tao Chi Kung practices have been refined and changed for thousands of years. There is nothing wrong with experimenting with new ways of doing things, provided that the experimentation is done in a responsible way. If you want to change the practice in some way, discuss it first with the person or people who trained you. Make sure your clients are aware that you want to try something new with them and they have given you formal consent to proceed before doing so.

The following are some guidelines to keep in mind as you consider helping other people with this approach.

HEAL YOURSELF FIRST

Once people become aware of how they can heal they often want to help others. However, in order to help someone to the maximum benefit, it is important that the helpers heal themselves first. One reason for that is that the energy of the helper will affect the person who is going through the procedure. If there is toxic energy in a helper, it will affect the field surrounding the person who is trying to heal.

Another reason is that the unresolved issues inside the helper may bias his or her perspective on how the afflicted person needs to heal and could lead the helper to give improper guidance. For example, if someone who has unresolved abuse issues tries to help someone who is trying to heal from those kinds of issues, he or she might view forgiveness differently than someone who does not have that history or those emotional wounds. That could lead the helper to steer the person away from forgiveness or to bring doubt into the process.

KEEP YOUR EGO OUT OF IT

Anyone who attempts to guide someone else through this process needs to make sure that he or she is doing so for the right reasons. If any part of the agenda is to make the person be impressed with how smart or powerful the guide is, that obscures the reality that the power of this approach comes from the process, not the person. It also affects the energetic field that surrounds the person who is trying to heal and may impede the healing process as a result.

TONGUE FU

An important aspect of effectively addressing the energetic residue of our pasts is realizing how we get caught up in vicious cycles and paradoxes. However, people vary in their willingness and ability to recognize how those factors have contributed to their condition. Therefore, as a guide, it is important to offer your observations, theories, and suggestions in a tentative way.

First, even if someone seems to have asked your opinion about her or his situation, it still might be helpful to ask if you can offer some feedback before you say it. When someone says "no" to that question, honor that. Prove through your behavior that your intention is about helping rather than showing how right you are. If the person says "yes," then he or she will be more open to whatever you have to say just by virtue of the fact that his or her answer invited your feedback. In other words, agreeing to receive feedback makes it easier for the person to accept it.

It is also important to leave room for doubt. Even if you are convinced that you are right, that does not mean that you are. Besides, offering your feedback in a tentative way makes it easier for the recipient to consider it. It does not seem like an accusation, just an observation for consideration. Starting your feedback with phrases like "It seems like . . ." "It appears that . . ." and "I wonder if . . ." will make your feedback feel more like an invitation for discussion rather than a statement of fact that cannot be disputed. Be aware that just because something has worked for you does not mean it will necessarily work the same way for someone else.

Be prepared to have a session or two just talking with some people who come to you for help. You cannot be certain that everyone you meet will be ready to trust the treatment process enough to jump right into it.

OPEN QUESTIONS

In order to help people sort out what topic and what aspects of the topic they should focus on in the exercise it is helpful to use open questions. Closed questions are the type that can easily be responded to with a "yes" or "no." Examples of closed questions are "Do you want to focus on your childhood?" or "Did your Dad do that to you?" As you can probably tell, those types of questions can lead people to feel restricted in what they are allowed to think about and can even seem to be making suggestions instead of asking questions.

Open questions are more difficult to answer with a "yes" or "no" response and they tend to start with "Who," "What," "When," and "Where." "Why" is not usually used because it too often puts people on the defensive. Examples of open questions that you could use to help someone sort out what to focus on in this exercise are:

What experiences have you had that still bother you now and you wish
they didn't?

What comes to mind when you think about that issue?

What negative belief have you concluded about yourself because of
that issue?

How much does the issue (still) affect you when you think about it now?

Where do you feel a reaction in your body when you think about it?

REFLECTING SKILLS

People often fear being judged or misunderstood if they reveal negative
experiences from their pasts. Using reflecting skills can help to reassure
them that you understand and are not judging their histories. Whenever someone asks you something like "Do you know what I mean?"
that is a cue to start using this type of communication skill. Reflecting
skills can be broken down into three parts:

1. Say what the person has said to you in your own words.
2. Say why you think the person has brought up that topic or
   aspect of the topic.
3. Ask "Am I right?"

For example, a person you are helping might say to you, "I'm such
an idiot for letting that happen to me." Using reflecting skills, you
would resist the temptation to react to that statement and instead say
something like "You blame yourself because you think that there was
something that you could have done that would have prevented it from
happening. Am I right?"

The three-part structure of reflecting skills helps to ensure that you
convey to the person you are helping that you are trying to understand
and that you are not coming to any definite conclusions about the situation without first checking your perceptions with him or her. Do not
be discouraged if it takes several uses of reflecting skills before the per-

son agrees that you understand him or her completely. Continuing to make genuine attempts only proves that you are determined to understand without judging or jumping to conclusions.

Some Procedural Tips: Checking In

1. Between each set, ask the person what happened.
2. Listen and watch for signs that the person is getting sore eyes, too tired, or too upset.
3. Give lots of permission for the person to share any discomfort and to take whatever measures are needed to make the process manageable.
4. Check periodically with the person about whether he or she wants guidance from you about when to start and stop each type of eye movement. After a while some people want to decide that part on their own.
5. Validate and normalize the reactions the person has while doing the processing. Offer reassurance that it is typical to have confusing thoughts, images, feelings, and body reactions.
6. Avoid talking a lot to explain the reactions that a person is having during the treatment. Save that kind of discussion for the end of the session. Otherwise you could end up spending time talking and giving information that the person could have used to heal.

If the Person Gets Stuck or Overwhelmed

If the person gets overwhelmed in the process, take a break and lead him or her through the Inner Smile, Microcosmic Orbit, or Six Healing Sounds to help the person feel calm and centered.

If the person cannot let go of the negative feelings connected to the issue that is being addressed after several attempts then you could:

1. Bring the person back to the first image that was used to access the issue and start processing from there again.

2. Focus on the body sensations and try to process them first before going back to the images and beliefs about the issue.

3. Offer a new way of looking at the situation and have the person focus on that as you start the next round of processing.

BRINGING IN OTHER UNIVERSAL HEALING TAO PRACTICES

Cosmic Healing Connection

People who have Taoist Cosmic Healing training can add some vital energy to the healing process. You can also tap on your client's legs to facilitate the processing, but be mindful that your energy will be interacting with the person you are trying to help. Make sure your energy is clean and strong before you try to help someone else this way. Pass energy through your palms to the person as you tap (fig. 9.1).

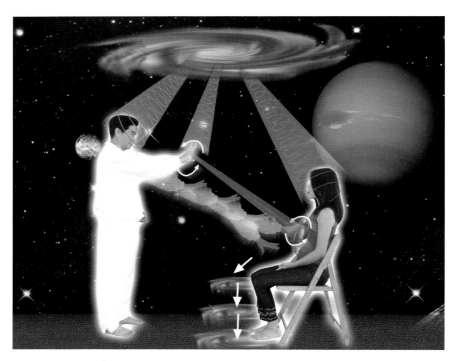

Fig. 9.1. Combining Taoist Emotional Recycling with Taoist Cosmic Healing

CHI NEI TSANG AND BODY DIAGNOSIS

If you are a certified practitioner in Chi Nei Tsang your diagnostic skills can help in this treatment. You can use them to help your clients figure out where to focus in the last section of the exercise in which you clean up any leftover negative energy that is stored in the body. You can look at their tongues, eyes, skin, hair, nails, and navels. You can also feel for heat or toxic energy coming off the body, take their wrist pulses, and check their other body pulses.

This practice and Chi Nei Tsang fit well together. You can alternate between the two for maximum benefit for your clients. For example, you may help clients transform the negative energy around an issue, then work on their energy systems manually using Chi Nei Tsang while they focus on the issue, and then go back to this method to make sure there are no other leftover emotions, beliefs, or physical discomforts that have cropped up after doing Chi Nei Tsang with them.

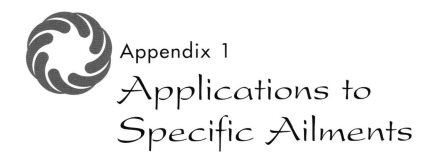

Appendix 1
Applications to Specific Ailments

 ## Neglect

Deciding what to focus on when the issue that you have chosen has to do with neglect can be tricky because neglect involves the absence of something happening. However, you can still do it. Try focusing on the location where the neglect occurred. For example, if you believe that your parents neglected you, you could start by picturing a room in your family home.

 ## Hyperactivity

Your diaphragm overlaps most of your internal organs. When we get stressed it tends to pull tight and does not always release after the stress has passed. If it stays tight it can restrict all of your internal organs and therefore affect your emotional state. It can also lead to a lot of heat being trapped in the top half of your upper body, which can contribute to hyperactivity.

Concentrate on your diaphragm muscle and do the eye and/or hand movements after you have treated all of your internal organs.

Addictions

1. Identify the people, places, and situations (commonly referred to as "triggers") that seem to impel you to use something addictive. More than one trigger may come up in the process, which may quicken the healing process. If there are other triggers that did not come up in the first round of processing, they can be addressed as separate topics after completing the process with the first trigger.
2. Any shame or guilt you feel as a result of having an addiction should be targeted as a specific trigger.
3. Triggers can be positive, too. Target the most pleasurable experiences you had in the past with your addiction to relieve their pull on you to resume the addictive substance or activity.

 Phobias

1. Make a list of all the different versions of the object or situation that you fear. Rank them from least frightening to most frightening.
2. Then address each version, one at a time, using the procedure, starting with the least frightening and working your way systematically to the most frightening scenario.

 Pain

Many physical pains are created by or made worse by emotional conditions.

1. Make a list of all the situations in which your pain feels worse.
2. Then rank those situations from the ones that lead to the least amount of increased pain to the ones that make it the worst.
3. Then focus on each situation, one at a time, and go through the entire procedure, starting with the situation that leads to the least amount of increased pain and progressing systematically to the situation that creates the most amount of pain for you.
4. You can also focus directly on the painful area and do the processing.

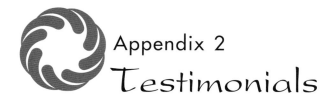

Appendix 2
Testimonials

My name is Orlando Canages. I am fifty-four years old. I grew up in El Salvador. I have lived in British Columbia for twenty-four years now. I fled from El Salvador to get away from the pressure to take a side and join the Twelve-Years War in my country. After I moved to Canada, though, I found that I still was affected by what had happened around me in my country. I had flashbacks and nightmares about the war. At times I would react to loud noises as if I were about to be attacked. One time I remember walking down a street and a car backfired. I hit the ground. I thought someone was shooting at me. The people around me were all standing and looking at me. I started drinking to forget my past. At one point I was drinking a full twenty-six-ounce bottle of alcohol every night.

Many people suggested that I should go for counseling but I did not want to do that. Many of my friends had gone to counseling for the same issues; some of them had gone for years, but they did not seem to be getting any better. When Doug approached me about doing Taoist Emotional Recycling I did not know what to expect, but I soon found out that this approach was a lot different. When we started processing the emotions while focusing on the forehead I felt the emotions going away quickly. Within a few sets I felt totally relaxed. I felt like I was going to go to sleep. We only worked for a half hour but I already felt a lot better. Doug taught me how to keep working on my own until the next session. I tried it a couple of times and was able to completely get rid of the feelings connected to that issue. It just felt like the issue was getting further and further away from me every time I worked on it.

In the next session Doug explained that we were going to start working on the internal organs and why that is important. I didn't know what to expect. We worked on the heart and spleen and I didn't get much of a reaction other than an increasing sense of peace inside. Working on the lungs was a different story, though. In the first set of working on the lungs I got an emotional reaction of sadness and grief that was so strong that I couldn't stop it from pouring out of me. It was a like an explosion. We talked about how that made sense given that the lungs are connected to grief and sadness. It only took two more sets to completely clear that emotion away. Then we moved on to the kidneys. Again I felt a strong emotional reaction during the processing, but not as strong as it had been with the lungs. Doug explained that the kidneys are connected to fear and anxiety, so it made sense to me why I got another reaction in that area. I'm really amazed at how quickly and how well this technique works. I'm grateful that I've been able to benefit from it.

Ever since I walked through Doug Hilton's door to seek help for the crippling issues I had been dealing with my life has been forever changed. In the past I had sought out many different mental health professionals of all walks and never achieved the results I gained after seeing Doug. After a few sessions, Doug suggested a very different concept and approach to helping me overcome the barriers that had really stunted my quality of life.

Doug was able to explain the theory and process in a way that was really interesting and intriguing. Even though I didn't know what to expect, or how it could actually work, my faith in Doug was already there. So after some very simple questions Doug created a plan to execute this amazing process and we dove in. The process was very simple and easy to do. We focused on the issue, starting with the heart. As we went through the different organs I could feel the difference in the impact to my body. Sometimes it was very intense and in other organs not so much. Some of it was surprising! Using EMDR previously had been very useful, but this time, it was like the layers were being pulled back and with the circular motion of the eyes I perceived it as flushing the toxic feelings down the drain. I also noticed that I did not feel exhausted after the session like I did after EMDR. To be honest, it was so easy that while we were using the technique I really wasn't sure anything was happening. We finished our session and Doug coached me on doing this process by myself, which was very helpful, because I could deal with issues as I felt or remembered them. I left hopeful but with some skepticism.

I am no longer a skeptic! Since my sessions I have noticed that these long-standing issues that we worked on and the powerful feelings connected with them have become lessened to almost nothing. That is not to say I felt numb, or forgot the experience, or the things I had learned from the traumatic events; rather they had become manageable thoughts to reflect on. No longer did these memories invoke panic attacks, full blown meltdowns, and the inability to get on with my day. Now what brings me to tears is how grateful I am to Doug for helping me and showing me how to release myself from the "prison" I had been living in every single day. I sincerely recommend to anyone who is looking for a new way and a new lease on life to seek the Taoist Emotional Recycling technique therapy.

DENA ESARY

I did EMDR with Doug in the past, so I thought I had some idea what to expect when he offered to show me Taoist Emotional Recycling. The experience was different from what I noticed when we did EMDR, though. This time Doug only offered a short explanation and explained other parts of how the technique worked as we went along. When we did EMDR there was a long explanation at the beginning. There were no preliminary exercises or a set of questions to answer at the beginning, either. Like EMDR, the process worked. After it was over I did not feel any emotion connected to the issue I chose at all. However, the process was faster. Altogether it took about an hour to do all the steps of the new technique. While we were doing it I didn't have a bunch of other memories or feelings come up like I did when we used EMDR, but the other memories that were connected to the issue seemed to be dealt with anyway. I wasn't tired at the end of the process like I was when we did EMDR. I went right back to work afterward and I was fine. The only reaction I noticed that seemed unusual was that I was sweating a lot on my back at one point.

The issue I was working on is an ongoing one. It's still happening in my life. However, after addressing it with the technique I don't feel as angry when the issue comes up. The experiences that I addressed using Taoist Emotional Recycling have not come back since we worked on them. Doug taught me how to do the technique on my own at the end of the session. I've been able to do that a couple of times already and I'm confident that I could apply it to other issues in my life.

TINA WONG

My name is Selina Su. I have never had any kind of counseling before. When Doug asked me to try Taoist Emotional Recycling I didn't know what was going to happen. He explained the process for a few minutes. It seemed to make sense. He asked me to choose a topic to focus on, something from my past that still bothers me. I picked an issue that had bothered me for a couple of years. For some reason that issue still really bothered me, even though the person it involved isn't in my life anymore.

When we went through the steps in the technique it seemed like a long process to me, but not complicated. At the end of the hour the issue didn't bother me at all. I was calm and had energy. I went home that night and looked at pictures of the person that I had focused on when I did the treatment. That hardly bothered me at all. I didn't even focus on those pictures of her when we did the process. Doug taught me how to do the technique on my own and suggested that I focus on those pictures or any other issues that are connected to the issue we worked on that did not get completely worked out the first time. I know how to do the technique now and will do that if I need to, but so far it doesn't seem necessary.

Doug offered to show my husband and me a new technique for putting away bad feelings about things that happened in the past. We were willing to see what that was about.

He gave us a quick introduction to what we were going to do and then we quickly got to work on dealing with the issue we chose. We both chose the same issue because it affected both of us and still bothered us both. We started the processing in the forehead and the emotion around that issue quickly went away. I (Miranda) got a bit of a headache. Doug gave me some water and explained that the heat that is created from moving the energy sometimes gives people headaches at first. The headache went away. Then we worked on the heart. That seemed easy enough. We both felt peaceful and good after we worked there. When we worked on the spleen that was a different story. We both reacted to that one. Doug explained that the spleen can be connected to worry, overthinking, and negative thinking. I have the tendency to overthink things and Robert has a tendency to worry, so it made sense to us that we would have more of a reaction when we worked there.

At the end of the session Doug let us know how we could use what he showed us on our own. It seemed simple enough. We will try it when we get upset about something in the future.

Miranda and Robert Doig

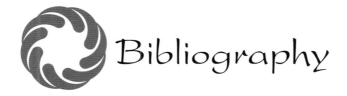 Bibliography

Chia, Mantak. *Chi Nei Tsang*. Rochester, Vt.: Destiny Books, 2007.

———. *Chi Self-Massage*. Rochester, Vt.: Destiny Books, 2006.

———. *Cosmic Detox*. Rochester, Vt.: Destiny Books, 2011.

———. *Healing Light of the Tao*. Rochester, Vt.: Destiny Books, 2008.

———. *Healing Love through the Tao*. Rochester, Vt.: Destiny Books, 2005.

———. *The Inner Smile*. Rochester, Vt.: Destiny Books, 2008.

———. *Sexual Reflexology*. Rochester, Vt.: Destiny Books, 2003.

———. *The Six Healing Sounds*. Rochester, Vt.: Destiny Books, 2009.

———. *Tan Tien Chi Kung*. Rochester, Vt.: Destiny Books, 2004.

———. *Taoist Cosmic Healing*. Rochester, Vt.: Destiny Books, 2003.

Chia, Mantak, and Lee Holden. *Simple Chi Kung*. Rochester, Vt.: Destiny Books, 2011.

Chia, Mantak, and Tao Huang. *The Secret Teachings of the Tao Te Ching*. Rochester, Vt.: Destiny Books, 2005.

Chia, Mantak, and William U. Wei. *Chi Kung for Prostate Health and Sexual Vitality*. Rochester, Vt.: Destiny Books, 2013.

———. *Chi Kung for Women's Health and Sexual Vitality*. Rochester, Vt.: Destiny Books, 2014.

Davis, Ronald D. *The Gift of Dyslexia*. San Francisco: Ability Workshop Press, 1994.

Emoto, Masaru. *The Miracle of Water*. New York: Atria Books, 2007.

Hilton, Doug V. "Polarities, Gestalts and Metapsychology." Master's thesis. University of Calgary, 1994.

Lerner, Harriet. *The Dance of Deception*. New York: HarperCollins, 1993.

Lipton, Bruce. *The Biology of Belief*. Carlsbad, Calif.: Hay House, 2008.

Miller, Robert. "The Feeling-State Theory of Behavioral and Substance Addictions and the Feeling-State Addiction Protocol." 2011. www .psychinnovations.com/EMDRSD/Miller_Feeling_State_Addiction .pdf [accessed July 13, 2013].

Mitchell, Stephen, trans. *Tao Te Ching.* New York: Harper Perennial, 1991.

Pearsall, Paul. *The Heart's Code.* New York: Random House, 1998.

Schwartz, Gary. E., with William L. Simon. *The Energy Healing Experiments.* New York: Atria Books, 2007.

Siegel, Daniel. J. *The Mindful Brain.* New York: W. W. Norton & Company, 2007.

What the Bleep Do We Know?! DVD. Directed by W. Arntz, B. Chasse, and M. Vicente Fox. Los Angeles: Roadside Attractions, 2004.

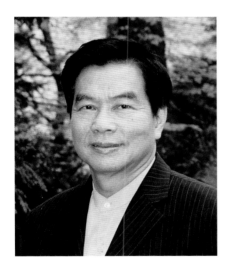

About the Authors

MANTAK CHIA

Mantak Chia has been studying the Taoist approach to life since childhood. His mastery of this ancient knowledge, enhanced by his study of other disciplines, has resulted in the development of the Universal Healing Tao system, which is now being taught throughout the world.

Mantak Chia was born in Thailand to Chinese parents in 1944. When he was six years old, he learned from Buddhist monks how to sit and "still the mind." While in grammar school he learned traditional Thai boxing, and he soon went on to acquire considerable skill in aikido, yoga, and Tai Chi. His studies of the Taoist way of life began in earnest when he was a student in Hong Kong, ultimately leading to his mastery of a wide variety of esoteric disciplines, with the guidance of several masters, including Master I Yun, Master Meugi, Master Cheng Yao Lun, and Master Pan Yu. To better understand the mechanisms behind healing energy, he also studied Western anatomy and medical sciences.

Master Chia has taught his system of healing and energizing practices to tens of thousands of students and trained more than two thousand instructors and practitioners throughout the world. He has established centers for Taoist study and training in many countries around the globe. In 1990 and in 2012, he was honored by the International Congress of Chinese Medicine and Qi Gong (Chi Kung), which named him the Qi Gong Master of the Year.

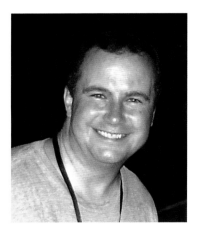

DOUG HILTON

Doug Hilton is a Universal Healing Tao instructor and practitioner. He is also a psychotherapist in private practice in Burnaby, British Columbia, Canada. In his career as a psychotherapist, spanning more than twenty years, Doug has worked with children, teens, adults, and seniors. He has worked specifically with psychiatric conditions, trauma, and addictions. If you want to know more about Doug's services you can check out his website at www.fullcirclehealing.ca.

The Universal Healing Tao System and Training Center

THE UNIVERSAL HEALING TAO SYSTEM

The ultimate goal of Taoist practice is to transcend physical boundaries through the development of the soul and the spirit within the human. That is also the guiding principle behind the Universal Healing Tao, a practical system of self-development that enables individuals to complete the harmonious evolution of their physical, mental, and spiritual bodies. Through a series of ancient Chinese meditative and internal energy exercises, the practitioner learns to increase physical energy, release tension, improve health, practice self-defense, and gain the ability to heal him- or herself and others. In the process of creating a solid foundation of health and well-being in the physical body, the practitioner also creates the basis for developing his or her spiritual potential by learning to tap into the natural energies of the sun, moon, earth, stars, and other environmental forces.

The Universal Healing Tao practices are derived from ancient techniques rooted in the processes of nature. They have been gathered and integrated into a coherent, accessible system for well-being that works directly with the life force, or chi, that flows through the meridian system of the body.

Master Chia has spent years developing and perfecting techniques for teaching these traditional practices to students around the world through ongoing classes, workshops, private instruction, and healing sessions, as well as books and video and audio products. Further information can be obtained at www.universal-tao.com.

THE UNIVERSAL HEALING TAO TRAINING CENTER

The Tao Garden Resort and Training Center in northern Thailand is the home of Master Chia and serves as the worldwide headquarters for Universal Healing Tao activities. This integrated wellness, holistic health, and training center is situated on eighty acres surrounded by the beautiful Himalayan foothills near the historic walled city of Chiang Mai. The serene setting includes flower and herb gardens ideal for meditation, open-air pavilions for practicing Chi Kung, and a health and fitness spa.

The center offers classes year round, as well as summer and winter retreats. It can accommodate two hundred students, and group leasing can be arranged. For information on courses, books, products, and other Universal Healing Tao resources, see below.

RESOURCES

Universal Healing Tao Center
274 Moo 7, Luang Nua, Doi Saket, Chiang Mai, 50220 Thailand
Tel: (66)(53) 495-596 Fax: (66)(53) 495-852
E-mail: universaltao@universal-tao.com
Web site: www.universal-tao.com

For information on retreats and the health spa, contact:
Tao Garden Health Spa & Resort
E-mail: info@tao-garden.com, taogarden@hotmail.com
Web site: www.tao-garden.com

Good Chi • Good Heart • Good Intention

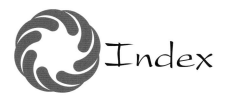

Index

Numbers in *italics* indicate illustrations.

BOOKS OF RELATED INTEREST

The Art of Cosmic Vision
Practices for Improving Your Eyesight
by Mantak Chia and Robert T. Lewanski

Basic Practices of the Universal Healing Tao
An Illustrated Guide to Levels 1 through 6
by Mantak Chia and William U. Wei

Craniosacral Chi Kung
Integrating Body and Emotion in the Cosmic Flow
by Mantak Chia and Joyce Thom

Healing Light of the Tao
Foundational Practices to Awaken Chi Energy
by Mantak Chia

Chi Self-Massage
The Taoist Way of Rejuvenation
by Mantak Chia

The Six Healing Sounds
Taoist Techniques for Balancing Chi
by Mantak Chia

Healing Love through the Tao
Cultivating Female Sexual Energy
by Mantak Chia

Pi Gu Chi Kung
Inner Alchemy Energy Fasting
by Mantak Chia and Christine Harkness-Giles

INNER TRADITIONS • BEAR & COMPANY
P.O. Box 388
Rochester, VT 05767
1-800-246-8648
www.InnerTraditions.com

Or contact your local bookseller